Anti-Inflammatory Cookbook 2021:

Over 100 Delicious Recipes to Reduce Inflammation, Be Healthy and Feel Amazing

Felicia Renolds

Table of Contents

Introduction

Congratulations on purchasing the *Anti-inflammatory Complete 2021: Over 100 Delicious Recopies To Reduce Inflammation, Be Healthy and Feel Amazing* and thank you for doing so. Deciding to change your diet for the better is a big step and one you should be applauded for making. It is also the easiest step; however, making a true lifestyle change requires commitment and dedication to ensure your new actions stick around long enough to become habits.

Having plenty of choices when it comes to healthy recipes choices is a big part of forming those new habits successfully, which is why the following chapters will provide you with plenty of choices regardless of what type of delicious and nutritious recipe you are looking for. Remember, before starting any new diet, it is important to check with a dietitian or your primary healthcare provider to ensure you don't accidentally end up doing more harm than good.

With so many choices out there when it comes to consuming this type of content, it is appreciated that you've chosen this one. Plenty of care and effort went into ensuring it contains as many interesting and useful tidbits as possible; please enjoy!

Chapter 1: Anti-Inflammatory Diet Rundown

As the name implies, the anti-inflammation diet is a loose collection of rules related to dietary choices designed to reduce the amount of negative chronic inflammation known to lead to everything from arthritis, cancer, and even death. Inflammation is not all bad; however, it can help the body defend against possible infection and heal cuts and wounds when it occurs naturally in the body.

Suppose it continues for a prolonged period of time. In that case, however, it can lead to a host of illnesses and other negative effects (described in detail in chapter 2), some of which can cause serious long term consequences when left unchecked. Luckily, there are numerous easy ways to reduce your levels of overall inflammation, including changing your eating habits, which is where the anti-inflammatory diet comes into play.

As a part of the inflammation process, the body creates an increased amount of immune cells, white blood cells and a substance known as cytokine to combat infection. There are two primary types of inflammation. The first is a short term variety that presents itself as swelling, heat, pain, and redness. This is the early phase of inflammation, and the symptoms that it brings along with it are caused by the fact that additional blood is flowing to the affected areas in an effort to treat the area as quickly as possible. This ensures that the troubled spot is protected from additional injury as the body works to fend off irritants, damaged cells, pathogens, viruses, and bacteria. Without the inflammation process, even minor cuts and wounds would never heal properly.

Alternately, chronic inflammation happens slowly over a period of months or years while outwardly presenting no noticeable signs of the ever-growing internal issue. This, in turn, creates a gradual shift in the types of cells that exist around the spot of the inflammation as the spot will constantly be in the process of destruction and rebirth, sapping bodily resources and slowly festering and becoming something much worse than whatever the initial injury may have been. This prolonged inflammation can be caused by numerous issues, including things like a failure to remove whatever caused the initial inflammation, a misfiring autoimmune response is attacking otherwise healthy cells or the continued presence of a low-level irritant. This will continue until, eventually, things get so bad in the inflamed area that the loss of function of a related vital process begins to occur.

What to Do About It

Unfortunately, the average diet of most of the Western world does little to combat chronic inflammation while at the same time doing plenty to help it along. This includes things like a distinct lack of omega-3 fatty acids as they are rarely found in the processed food that is growing increasingly more prevalent worldwide. Unfortunately, these processed foods do contain a large amount of omega-6 fatty acids, and this imbalance specifically is known to cause an increase in the amount of inflammation that a person experiences. What's worse, the lengths that most people have to go to on a regular basis to ensure they are eating nutritious foods that have not been processed makes it difficult for them to do so regularly.

This is where the anti-inflammatory diet comes in as it makes it easier for individuals to know that what they are eating is actively reducing the inflammatory buildup that they have been experiencing for years prior to the switch. A big reason for this is phytochemicals, naturally occurring chemicals that are found in many of the foods suggested in chapter 3 which are all known to reduce inflammation to various degrees.

Increasing the amount of omega-3 fatty acids that they consume on a regular basis is known to have an even greater benefit for those with rheumatoid arthritis, as consuming more than 3 grams each day has been directly shown to decrease the amount of stiffness, swollenness, and tenderness seen in affected joints. It is also known to have a notable impact on osteoarthritis pain for the same reasons.

A healthy example of a 24-hour anti-inflammation meal plan can be something as simple as steel-cut oatmeal topped with berries or yogurt as well as c of green tea or even coffee. For lunch, a tuna salad sandwich on whole grain bread along with a seasonal fruit smoothie. An afternoon snack could consist of something like walnuts and a bit of dark chocolate, and dinner could be whole grain pasta with an organic tomato sauce and turkey meatballs along with a salad made with walnuts, oranges, and spinach. The day could then be topped with a cranberry and apple pie that avoids the use of coconut oil.

While the primary use for the diet isn't weight loss, the focus on natural, healthy meals with reasonable portion sizes means that many individuals do experience a degree of weight loss. This is especially true when it comes to those who previously consumed a higher than average amount of processed foods. This is a naturally occurring phenomenon that comes about when a person decides to eat fewer carbohydrates, unhealthy oils, and trans fats while at the same time filling up on healthy alternatives instead, and there is no secret behind it; just clean, healthy eating.

With that being said, it is important to not expect too much too soon as the anti-inflammatory diet is always going to take longer to work than medicines designed directly to affect the problem in question. Rather, the anti-inflammatory diet is a positive lifestyle change that anyone can make that will, over time, make the need for such medicines completely unnecessary. The anti-inflammation diet won't change your level of inflammation overnight, but it will change it for good.

What to Eat and What to Avoid

When it comes to eating with an eye towards anti-inflammatory foods, there are plenty of options when it comes to avoiding the multitude of harmful products that contain inflammatory producing agents that can broadly be broken down into a handful of categories. Commit the following guidelines for the foods to eat and the foods to avoid to memory, and you will be inflammation free in no time flat.

Eat more fiber: Studies show that a diet that is high in fiber is naturally going to create an overall lower level of inflammation because of all of the phytonutrients that natural, unprocessed foods, including fruits and vegetables, have in spades. To ensure you consume 25 grams of fiber per day, make a point of eating lots of blueberries (3.5 grams), bananas (3 grams), onions, eggplant, okra, oatmeal, and barley.

Aim for 9 servings of vegetables and fruits every day: Make a point of consuming a ratio of 2 to 1 vegetables when compared to fruits as too many fruits in a single day can cause your total sugar intake to increase rapidly. A serving is generally considered half a c of cooked vegetables or 1 cup of raw vegetables. Both ginger and turmeric are known to fight inflammation as well, and both make great seasonings.

Aim for 4 servings of crucifers and alliums each week: Alliums are things like leeks, onions, scallions, and garlic, while crucifers comprise numerous vegetables, including Brussels sprouts, mustard greens, cauliflower, cabbage, and broccoli. These all contain extremely high levels of antioxidants, which is why only a few each week is enough to significantly lower your risk of inflammation-related cancer when consumed regularly. Remember, 4 servings a week is the minimum when it comes to alliums and crucifers. The more, the merrier.

Keep saturated fat to a minimum: In order to start actively reducing the amount of inflammation in your body, it is important that you start keeping a close eye on the number of saturated fats that you are consuming on a daily basis. This means cutting it to 10 percent of the total number of calories that you consume in a day. This means you will likely want to cut down on the red meat and stick with healthy marinates made from anti-inflammatory spices instead of Coconut oil.

Eat lots of omega-3 fatty acids: As previously discussed, eating more omega-3 fatty acids should be at the top of the list of anyone who is interested in decreasing their inflammation level. In addition to being found in fish, it is also found in large doses in walnuts, flaxseeds and soy, kidney and navy beans. A regular omega-3 supplement is also recommended. When it comes to fish, anchovies, sardines, trout, mackerel, herring, oysters and salmon all contain the highest amounts of omega-3 and you should aim to eat 3 of them each week.

Seek out healthy fats: Fats have gotten somewhat of a bad rap over the years because, at some point, mainstream society decided to start lumping all fats together. In truth, there are healthy fats, which are a good source of energy for those who eschew carbohydrates in favor of a more natural energy solution. This means that plenty of healthy fats like those found in coconut oil, coconut oil and pressed canola oil are a great way to eat healthy while still expelling inflammatory elements from your system.

Avoid products made with corn syrup and/or refined sugar: Studies show that simply adding a daily dose of processed foods to your diet by eating things that are dosed with high amounts of sugar or corn syrup is enough to increase your inflammation levels significantly. Unfortunately, processed food companies understand that the more sugar something has in it, the more likely it is to sell, which means that it is virtually impossible to find anything processed that has enough sugar or corn syrup in it to cause inflammation in at least 2 full-grown adults. This intense fructose overload is enough to cause inflammation in the lining of blood vessels and should be avoided whenever possible.

Avoid trans-fat: In addition to saturated fats, it is important to avoid trans-fats as often as possible. This means looking at product labels as trans-fats are often hiding under the label of partially hydrogenated oils. Trans-fats are known to cause inflammation in the cell lining of the arteries as well as lower beneficial cholesterol levels which increase that of the harmful variety.

Avoid the wrong types of oil: In general, the healthy fat-based oils that are listed above are a healthy option. All others should be avoided regardless of the health claims they may tout. These oils are often extracted using chemicals that are known to increase inflammation and are rarely disclosed on product labels as they are used in the creation of the product and not added in after the fact. What's more, they are also typically high in omega-6 fatty acids, decreasing the balance in the body between that and omega-3 fatty acids and increasing inflammation in the process.

Avoid refined carbohydrates: While complex carbohydrates are a great source of energy, refined carbohydrates are typically simple carbohydrates, which means they break down extremely quickly while also being responsible for the low energy feeling related to a sugar crash. What's more, the refining process is simply another word for the processing, which means they are stripped of what little nutritional value that they would otherwise have. They are also typically high in sugar, which makes them a trigger for inflammation in just about every possible way imaginable.

Avoid too much alcohol: When consumed to excess, both beer and hard alcohol have been linked to an increase in inflammation if used regularly. A good rule of thumb is that men should stick with no more than 2 drinks per day, and women should limit themselves to 1 drink if they want to drink while at the same time keep their inflammation levels to a minimum.

Chapter 2: Breakfast Recipes

Anti-Inflammatory Blueberry Smoothie

Makes enough for 1
Time required for proper preparation: 5 minutes
Suggested cooking time: 0 minutes
Total required: 5 minutes

What to Use
Cayenne pepper (.25 tsp.)
- frozen banana (1)
- frozen blueberries (.5 c)
- cinnamon (.25 tsp)
- Maca powder (1 tsp.)
- almond Coconut oil (1 T)
- water (.5)
- spinach or leafy greens (2 handfuls)
- unsweetened almond milk (.5 c)

What to Do
- Add everything to a food processor or blender and blend/process until your desired consistency is reached

Cherry Coconut Porridge

Makes enough for 1
Time required for proper preparation: 10 minutes
Suggested cooking time: 5minutes
Total required: 15 minutes

What to Use
- Maple syrup (as desired)
- Dark chocolate flakes (as desired)
- Cherries (as desired)
- Coconut shavings (as desired)
- Stevia (1 pinch)
- Cacao (3 T raw)
- Coconut milk (3.5 c)
- Chia seed (4 T)
- Oats (5 c)

What to Do
- In a saucepan, add the stevia, cacao, coconut milk, chia, and oats together before placing the pan on the stove over a burner turned to medium heat.
- Let the mixture boil before turning the heat to low and letting everything simmer until the oats are completely cooked.
- Pour the results into a bowl, add the remaining ingredients as desired and serve hot

Goat Cheese/Zucchini Frittata

Makes enough for 4
Time required for proper preparation: 10 minutes
Suggested cooking time: 15 minutes
Total required: 25 minutes

What to Use
- Goat cheese (2 oz.)
- Garlic (1 clove)
- Coconut oil (1 T)
- Pepper (as desired)
- Salt (.25 tsp.)
- Milk (2 T)
- Eggs (8)
- Zucchinis (2 sliced)

What to Do
- Ensure your oven is preheated to 350F.
- Combine the pepper, salt, milk, and eggs together in a large bowl.
- Coat a pan in the oil and place it on the stove above a burner that has been turned to a high/medium heat.
- Add in the zucchini and garlic and let them sauté for approximately 5 minutes or until done.
- Add in the eggs and stir well for 60 seconds.
- Remove the pan from the stove, top frittata with cheese and bake for approximately 11 minutes.
- Let it cool for 3 minutes, serve warm and enjoy.

Tomato Frittata

Makes enough for 2
Time required for proper preparation: 15 minutes
Suggested cooking time: 10 minutes
Total required: 25 minutes

What to Use
- Halved cherry tomatoes (8)
- Chopped zucchini (1)
- Coconut oil (2 T)
- Pepper
- Salt
- Almond milk (.5 c.)
- Egg whites (3)
- Eggs (3)
- Grated Parmesan cheese (.25 c.)

What to Do
- Heat up the broiler of the oven to high, and move the rack of the oven to the middle.
- Take out a bowl and whisk together the pepper, salt, almond milk, egg whites, and eggs.
- In a skillet, heat up some coconut oil. Let it warm up until it starts to shimmer.
- Add in the tomatoes and the zucchini and cook for about five minutes, stirring a bit.
- Pour in your egg mixture to this and let everything cook for a bit. After four minutes, the edges should start to set.
- Using a spatula, you can pull the eggs away from the pan edges. Tilt the pan around so that the unset egg can make it on all the edges too.
- After another four minutes, you can sprinkle on the Parmesan cheese before transferring the pan to your broiler.
- Cook for three to five minutes, so the eggs have time to become puffy. Slice and serve.

Simple Chia Pudding

Makes enough for 4
Time required for proper preparation: 5 minutes
Suggested cooking time: 6 hours
Total required: 6 hours and 5 minutes

What to Use
- Extract (Vanilla) (1 tsp)
- Agave (1-2 T)
- Dairy-free milk (1.5 c)
- Chia seeds (0.5 c)

What to Do
- First, combine the maple syrup, vanilla extract, chia seeds, and dairy-free milk in a bowl. Then whisk the ingredients very well to mix them all together.
- Refrigerate the ingredients overnight or for at least 6 hours in the bowl (preferably overnight), so the chia pudding is thick and creamy. If the chia pudding is not thick and creamy, you can add more chia seeds. Then put it back into the refrigerator, and keep it in the refrigerator for about another hour or so until the pudding is firm. You can garnish it with fruit, almonds, or nuts of your choice.

Veggie Egg Muffins

Serves: 8
Time required for proper preparation: 20 minutes
Suggested cooking time: 30 minutes
Total required: 50 minutes

What to Use
- Onion (1 small, diced)
- Mushrooms (4 medium, sliced)
- Powdered garlic (2 tsp.)
- Salt (1 tsp.)
- Provolone cheese (.25 c shredded)
- Eggs (8)
- Milk (.25 c)
- Broccoli (2 c cut or torn into small florets)
- Bell pepper (1 c chopped)

What to Do
- Ensure your oven is heated to 350F.
- Grease the muffin pan, and fill with vegetables.
- In a large bowl, add the eggs, garlic powder & salt.
- Fill each c.75of the way with the egg mixture, then top with a pinch of cheese.
- Bake approximately 25 to 30 minutes or until puffy and golden brown.

Sweet Potato Breakfast Burrito

Makes enough for 1
Time required for proper preparation: 25 minutes
Suggested cooking time: 10 minutes
Total required: 35 minutes

What to Use
- Coconut oil (4 tsp.)
- Cheddar cheese (2 oz. shredded)
- Baby spinach (4 c packed, roughly chopped)
- Sweet potatoes (2 small peeled and diced)
- Yellow onions (2 small, chopped)
- Tricolor bell peppers (1.5 c frozen, sliced, thawed)
- 10-inch whole wheat tortillas (8)
- Chili powder (2 tsp.)
- Eggs (4 large beaten)
- Egg whites (4 large, beaten)

What to Do
- Place your skillet on the stove over a burner turned to medium heat. Sauté potato, onion and bell peppers for approximately 7 minutes. Toss in chili powder, spinach, and sauté for another 2 minutes.
- Increase the heat slightly to high/medium. Mix in eggs and egg whites. Cook for 3 minutes, continuing to stir until eggs are cooked completely and not runny. Remove from heat and cool for 10 minutes.
- Cut 8 16-inch pieces of aluminum foil. Place 1 tortilla on top of each piece. Put an equal portion of the egg mixture in the middle of each tortilla. Sprinkle cheese on top. Fold two sides in first, and then roll forward from the top of the burrito. Make sure the foil is wrapped tightly around the burrito but not inside the roll if you will be microwaving it to reheat.
- Place burritos into a large plastic bag in the fridge. There are two ways to reheat. You can either bake the burrito on a cookie sheet in a 400-degree oven for 35 minutes or cook in the microwave for 2 minutes. Transfer the burrito to a paper bag with a pair of tongs, and you can bring it with you on the run.

Porridge

Makes enough for: 1
Time required for proper preparation: 5 minutes
Suggested cooking time: 5 minutes
Total required: 10 minutes

What to Use
- Salt (1 pinch)
- Coconut cream (4 T)
- Psyllium husk powder (1 pinch ground)
- Coconut flour (1 T)
- Egg (1)
- Coconut oil (1 oz.)

What to Do
- Place everything together in a small pan before placing the pan on the stove on top of a burner set to low heat.
- Stir the results continuously to encourage porridge to thicken. Continue stirring until your preferred thickness is reached.
- A small amount of coconut milk or a few berries (fresh or frozen) can also be added as desired.

Carrot Muffins

Makes enough for: 12
Time required for proper preparation: 20 minutes
Suggested cooking time: 15 minutes
Total required: 35 minutes

What to Use
- Ground nutmeg (.5 tsp.)
- Ground ginger (2 tsp.)
- Ground cinnamon (2 tsp.)
- Baking powder (1 tsp.)
- Baking soda (1 tsp.)
- Brown sugar (3 T)
- Old-fashioned oats (.5 c.)
- Whole-wheat flour (1 c.)
- Oat bran (1 c.)
- Cooking spray
- Raisins (.25 c.)
- Grated carrots (1.5 c.)
- Coconut oil (2 T)
- Egg (1)
- Honey (2 T)
- Almond milk (1.25 c.)
- Salt (.25 tsp.)

What to Do
- Ensure your oven is ready at 350F. Line two muffin tins with some paper liners, or use your cooking spray for this.
- Now take out a big bowl and whisk together the salt, nutmeg, ginger, cinnamon, baking powder, baking soda, brown sugar, oats, all the flours, and the oat bran. Set it to the side.
- In another bowl, whisk together the coconut oil, egg, honey, and almond milk.
- Add your dry ingredients and wet ingredients together and mix to just blend. The batter will be lumpy and have some flour streaks still in it, and that is fine.
- Fold in the raisins and the carrots at this time.
- Take the batter and fill up the muffin cup before placing it into the oven. After 15 minutes, the muffins should be done. Allow them time to cool down before serving.

Berry Smoothie Bowl

Makes enough for: 1
Time required for proper preparation: 5 minutes
Suggested cooking time: 0 minutes
Total required: 5 minutes

What to Use
- Protein powder (1 scoop)
- Almond milk (2-3 T (can substitute coconut milk))
- Sliced ripe banana (1 that is frozen)
- Organic Frozen mixed berries (1 big c)
- Seeds (Hemp and Chia) (1 T)
- Shreds of coconut (Unsweetened) (1 T)

What to Do
- Blend the berries and ripened banana together.
- Add the almond milk to the protein powder and blend both until the mixture is blended smoothly. You can top with chia seeds, hemp seeds, or shredded unsweetened coconut if you would like.
- You can also substitute any non-dairy milk if you do not like dairy milk. To take the recipe to another level, you can also substitute a green or white tea as well.

Omelet with Mushrooms

Makes enough for: 1
Time required for proper preparation: 5 minutes
Suggested cooking time: 10 minutes
Total required: 15 minutes

What to Use
- Mushrooms (3 chopped)
- Onion (.25 chopped)
- Sharp cheddar cheese (1 oz. shredded)
- Coconut oil (1 oz. grass fed)
- Pepper (as desired)
- Salt (as desired)

What to Do
- In a mixing bowl, add the eggs and season as desired before whisking well until the eggs become a batter.
- Add in a majority of the onion, mushroom as well as another pinch of salt to the mixing bowl, and mix well.
- Add the coconut oil to a frying pan before placing it on top of a burner set to a high/medium heat. Once the coconut oil is completely melted, add in the batter.
- Once the omelet begins to harden, top with the remaining onions and mushrooms before adding the cheese. With the help of a spatula, fold the egg on top of itself and continue cooking until it takes on a cooked, golden brown appearance.

Spinach Frittata with Bacon

Makes enough for: 4
Time required for proper preparation: 5 minutes
Suggested cooking time: 35 minutes
Total required: 40 minutes

What to Use
- Pepper (as desired)
- Salt (as desired)
- Coconut oil (2 T grass fed)
- Cheese (5 oz. shredded)
- Bacon (5 oz.)
- Spinach (.5 lbs. fresh)
- Heavy whipping cream (1 c)
- Eggs (8 large)

What to Do
- Start by making sure your oven is heated to 350F.
- Grease a baking dish using grass-fed Coconut oil.
- Add the coconut oil to a frying pan before placing it on the stove on top of a burner set to a medium/high heat before adding in the bacon and letting it fry until it reaches your desired level of crispiness, and then add in the spinach.
- Separately, mix together the cream and the eggs before whisking well.
- Add the results to the prepared baking dish before adding in the spinach and the bacon and topping with the shredded cheese.
- Place the dish in the oven for approximately 25 minutes. Let the frittata cool 5 minutes prior to removing it from baking dish.

Smoked Salmon Sammie on Pumpkin Bread

This recipe needs 5 minutes to prepare, 10 minutes to cook and will make 2 servings.

Makes enough for: 2
Time required for proper preparation: 5 minutes
Suggested cooking time: 10 minutes
Total required: 15 minutes

What to Use - Bread
- Coconut oil (1 T)
- Pumpkin puree (1 can)
- Coconut oil (.25 c)
- Apple sauce (.5 c unsweetened)
- Eggs (3 large)
- Pumpkin seeds (.3 c)
- Walnuts (.3 c chopped)
- Coconut flour (1.25 c)
- Almond flour (1.25 c)
- Flax seeds (.5 c)
- Psyllium husk (2 T powdered)
- Salt (1 tsp.)
- Baking powder (1 T)
- Pumpkin pie spice (2 T)

What to Use - Filling
- Chives (1 T chopped)
- Salmon (3 oz. smoked)
- Lettuce (1 oz.)
- Coconut oil (2 T grass fed)
- Chili flakes (1 pinch)
- Coconut oil (2 T grass fed)
- Pepper (as desired)
- Salt (as desired)
- Heavy whipping cream (2 T)
- Eggs (4 large)
- Egg (2 scrambled)

What to Do - Bread
- Start by making sure your oven is heated to 400F.
- Grease a bread pan (8 inches) using grass-fed Coconut oil
- In a large bowl, add the walnuts, coconut flour, almond flour, flax seeds, psyllium powder, salt, baking powder, and pumpkin pie spice and mix well.

- Mix in the pumpkin puree, coconut oil, apple sauce, and eggs and combine thoroughly.
- Add the batter to the prepared baking dish and top with 1 T pumpkin seeds.
- Place the pan on the bottom rack in the oven and let it bake for 60 minutes. You will know it is finished when you can stick a knife in, and it comes out clean.

What to Do - Sammie
- In a small bowl, combine the heavy whipping cream with the eggs and whisk well before seasoning as needed with pepper and salt.
- Add the coconut oil to a frying pan before placing in the stove on top of a burner set to medium heat. Once the coconut oil has melted, add in the egg mixture and stir well prior to removing the frying pan from the stove. Add in the chili powder and mix well
- Add the results to two pieces of toasted pumpkin bread, top with lettuce, smoked salmon, chives and scrambled eggs.

Scrambled Eggs with Avocado and Bacon

Makes enough for: 4
Time required for proper preparation: 2 minutes
Suggested cooking time: 10 minutes
Total required: 12 minutes

What to Use
- Pepper (as desired)
- Salt (as desired)
- Bacon (2 oz.)
- Coconut oil (1 tsp.)
- Avocado (.5 peeled)
- Eggs (2)

What to Do
- Preheat the oven to 350F.
- In a small pot, place the eggs and add cold water until the eggs are completely covered by roughly 1 inch of water. Add the pot to the stove above a boiler turned to a high/medium heat, and let the water boil.
- After the water has boiled, remove the pot from the stove, let it cool for roughly 10 minutes, and then drain the pot.
- Fill a large bowl with cold water and dunk the eggs briefly into it to make them easier to peel.
- Peel and prepare the eggs as preferred before placing them in a bowl; they should be warm, not hot.
- Split the eggs, remove the yolks, and discard them.
- In a large bowl, add the eggs, oil, and avocado and mix well before seasoning as desired.
- Place the bacon on a baking sheet and place the baking sheet in the oven for approximately 5 minutes or until done.
- Once the bacon is no longer hot to the touch, break each piece in half and portion out a half per serving of eggs.

Ham Omelet with Green Bell Peppers

Makes enough for: 2
Time required for proper preparation: 10 minutes
Suggested cooking time: 15 minutes
Total required: 25 minutes

What to Use
- Ham (5 oz. diced)
- Green bell pepper (.25 chopped fine)
- Onion (.5 yellow chopped fine)
- Coconut oil (2 oz. grass fed)
- Cheese (4 oz. shredded)
- Pepper (as desired)
- Salt (as desired)
- Sour cream (2 T)
- Eggs (6 large)

What to Do
- In a mixing bowl, combine the sour cream and eggs and whisk well before seasoning using salt and pepper as needed. Mix in 2 oz. shredded cheese.
- Add the coconut oil to a frying pan before placing the frying pan on the stove on top of a burner set to medium heat. Add in the onion, green pepper, and ham and let everything cook for 2 minutes, or the egg is nearly firm.
- Turn the burner to a low heat before adding the remaining cheese and folding the egg over on top of itself.

Egg Scramble

Makes enough for: 2
Time required for proper preparation: 10 minutes
Suggested cooking time: 15 minutes
Total required: 25 minutes

What to Use
- Pepper (as desired)
- Salt (as desired)
- Coconut oil (2 T)
- Olives (.5 c pitted)
- Parsley (.5 c chopped)
- Scallions (2)
- Halloumi cheese (4 oz. diced)
- Bacon (5 oz. diced)
- 5 eggs (large)

What to Do
- Add the oil to a frying pan before placing the pan on the stove on top of a burner set to medium heat. Add in the bacon, scallions, and halloumi and let it all brown.
- Combine the eggs and parsley in a small bowl and season as desired before whisking.
- Add the results to the pan before reducing the heat, adding in the olives and stir continuously for 2 additional minutes.

Grecian Breakfast Sandwich

Makes enough for: 2
Time required for proper preparation: 5 minutes
Suggested cooking time: 7 minutes
Total required: 12 minutes

What to Use
- Feta cheese (4 T)
- Tomato (1 sliced)
- Baby spinach (2 c)
- Eggs (4)
- Rosemary (1 T)
- Coconut oil (4 T)
- Multigrain sandwich thins (4)

What to Do
- Ensure your oven is preheated to 375F
- Brush the sandwich thins with coconut oil before adding them to a baking sheet and letting them bake for approximately 5 minutes or until done.
- Coat a pan in the oil and place it on the stove above a burner that has been turned to a high/medium heat.
- Add the eggs to the pan and let them cook for 60 seconds. Let the yolks break, and then flip the eggs and cook for an additional 60 seconds.
- Add all ingredients to sandwich thins, serve warm and enjoy.

Tabbouleh

Makes enough for: 4
Time required for proper preparation: 2 hours
Suggested cooking time: 0 minutes
Total required: 2 hours

What to Use
- Salt and pepper (as desired)
- Cucumber (1 peeled, seeded, chopped)
- Tomatoes (3 chopped)
- Mint (.25 c chopped)
- Parsley (1 c chopped)
- Green onions (1 c chopped)
- Lemon juice (.3 c)
- Coconut oil (.3 c)
- Water (1.5 c boiling)
- Bulgur (1 c)

What to Do
- Add the bulgur to the water, cover the pot and let it sit for 60 minutes.
- Mix in the cucumber, tomatoes, mint, parsley, onions, lemon juice, and oil before seasoning as needed.
- Add the lid back on and let it sit in the refrigerator for at least 60 minutes before serving.

Veggie Cakes

Makes enough for: 2
Time required for proper preparation: 10 minutes
Suggested cooking time: 15 minutes
Total required: 25 minutes

What to Use
- Salt and pepper (as desired)
- Walnuts (2 T chopped)
- Eggs (3 beaten)
- Sun-dried tomatoes (.25 c)
- Almond flour (.3 c)
- Kalamata olives (.3 c, sliced pitted)
- Artichoke hearts (.3 c)
- Parsnip (1 grated)
- Spinach (3 c)
- Garlic (3 cloves chopped)
- Onion (1 c chopped)
- Coconut oil (.25 c divided)

What to Do
- Coat a pan in half the oil and place it on the stove above a burner that has been turned to medium heat.
- Add in the garlic and onion and let them cook for approximately 5 minutes or until done.
- Add in the spinach and let it also cook for approximately 5 minutes or until done.
- Add the results to a large and let them cool.
- Into the bowl, add the remainder of the ingredients before combining well and forming the results into circles.
- Add the remainder of the oil to the pan and let the circles cook for approximately 5 minutes or until done per side.
- Serve hot and enjoy.

Cherry Coconut Porridge

Makes enough for: 1
Time required for proper preparation: 10 minutes
Suggested cooking time: 5 minutes
Total required: 15 minutes

What to Use
- Maple syrup (as desired)
- Dark chocolate flakes (as desired)
- Cherries (as desired)
- Coconut shavings (as desired)
- Stevia (1 pinch)
- Cacao (3 T raw)
- Coconut milk (3.5 c)
- Chia seed (4 T)
- Oats (5 c)

What to Do
- In a saucepan, add the stevia, cacao, coconut milk, chia, and oats together before placing the pan on the stove over a burner turned to medium heat.
- Let the mixture boil before turning the heat to low and letting everything simmer until the oats are completely cooked.
- Pour the results into a bowl, add the remaining ingredients as desired and serve hot.

Ginger, Apple Rhubarb Muffins

Makes enough for: 8
Time required for proper preparation: 15 minutes
Suggested cooking time: 20 minutes
Total required: 35 minutes

What to Use
- Salt (1 pinch)
- Ginger (.5 tsp. ground)
- Cinnamon (.5 tsp. ground)
- Baking powder (2 tsp. gluten-free)
- True arrowroot (2 T)
- Brown rice flour (.25 c)
- Buckwheat flour (.5 c)
- Linseed meal (1 T ground)
- Raw sugar (.25 c)
- Almonds (.5 c ground)
- Vanilla extract (1 tsp.)
- Egg (1 large)
- Coconut oil (.25 c)
- Rice milk (.3 c, 1 T)
- Apple (1 peeled, cored, diced)
- Rhubarb (1 c sliced)

What to Do
- Ensure your oven is heated to 350F.
- Coat a muffin tin in baking spray and add muffin liners.
- In a medium-sized bowl, mix together the linseed meal, ginger, sugar and almond meal.
- Mix the spices, flours and baking powder in evenly before adding the apple and rhubarb.
- In a separate bowl, add vanilla, egg, oil, and milk together before adding the results to the initial bowl.
- Add the batter to the tin, place the tin in the oven and let the muffins cook for 22 minutes. You will know they are finished when you can stick a toothpick into one of the muffins, and it comes out dry.
- Let the muffins cool before serving.

Chapter 3: Vegetarian Recipes

Hearts of Palm Black Bean Salad

Makes enough for: 2
Time required for proper preparation: 10 minutes
Suggested cooking time: 0 minutes
Total required: 10 minutes

What to Use
- Coconut oil (3 T)
- Vinegar (2 T)
- Parsley leaves (1 tsp fresh cut into small pieces)
- Jalapeño pepper (1 take out the seeds before using)
- Cilantro leaves (1 T cut into small pieces)
- Hearts of Palm (1 can)
- Lime juice (2 T)
- Chives (1 tsp fresh, cut into small pieces)
- Red onion (1 cut into thin slices)
- Black beans (1 c cooked according to package)
- Green onions (1 T)
- Corn (1 c cooked according to package)
- Yellow pepper (.5 c cut into thin slices)
- Avocado, (1 cut into small cubes)
- Pepper (as desired)
- Salt (as desired)

What to Do
- Using a mixing bowl, thoroughly combine vinegar, coconut oil, herbs, jalapeño, lime juice, salt, and Black pepper (as desired). Put to the side while preparing the salad.
- Cut the hearts of palm into .5 inch slices, making sure to cut at an angle.
- In another mixing bowl, mix the hearts of palm, black beans, red onions, corn, bell pepper, and green onions.
- When using for an appetizer, the mix can be served over greens. Add dressing over salad, top with avocado.

No-Noodle Lasagna

Makes enough for: 6
Time required for proper preparation: 10 minutes
Suggested cooking time: 1 hour 35 minutes
Total required: 1 hour 45 minutes

What to Use
- Spaghetti squash (1 large, ripe)
- Salt (as desired)
- Pepper (as desired)
- Marinara sauce (2 c)
- Ricotta (1 c)
- Parmesan cheese (8 tsp.)
- Mozzarella (6 oz. shredded)

What to Do
- Preheat oven to 375F.
- Cut the squash in half, and scoop out all the seeds and fibers with a spoon.
- Place on a baking sheet, with the cut side up, and season with the salt and pepper.
- Bake at 375F for about an hour or until the skin gives easily under pressure and the inside is tender. Remove from oven and let it cool for 10 minutes.
- Use a fork to create "noodles" from the squash. It will fluff up into spaghetti-like strands.
- Pour .25 c quick marinara sauce on the bottom of four individual 5 x 7-inch pans. Top the sauce with .75c of the spaghetti squash and spread evenly. Add .25 the total ricotta to each, top with mozzarella. Add mozzarella and bake for approximately 11 minutes.

Root Vegetable Casserole

Makes enough for: 4
Time required for proper preparation: 30 minutes
Suggested cooking time: 1 hour 30 minutes
Total required: 2 hours

What to Use
- Coconut oil (as needed)
- Heavy cream (1 c)
- Sour cream (6 T)
- Whole milk (1 c)
- Black pepper(as desired)
- Sea salt (as desired)
- Cheddar cheese (6 oz. grated)
- Celeriac (11 oz. halved, peeled, sliced thin)
- Turnips (13 oz. halved, peeled, sliced thin)
- Potatoes (1.5 lbs. halved, peeled, sliced thin)
- Rutabaga (1 lb. halved, peeled, sliced thin)

What to Do
- Ensure your oven is heated to 400F. Cover a baking dish (8x12) in coconut oil
- In a mixing bowl, combine the slices of celeriac, turnip, potatoes, and rutabaga together and mix well
- Place a saucepan on the stove on top of a burner set to a low heat before adding in the milk, sour cream and regular cream and mix until combined. Remove the saucepan from the burner and season using pepper as well as salt and stir repeatedly.
- Place half of the total amount of sliced root vegetables into a baking dish before seasoning and topping with a third of all of the cheese. Add a third of the total cream mixture to the top of the vegetables before adding in the rest of the vegetables and the rest of the cheese. Top with the rest of the cream.
- Place the results in the oven and let them bake for 90 minutes until the top is well-browned. Allow to cool and portion out into containers or plastic bags. This recipe can be refrigerated for 3-4 days or frozen for 2-3 months.

Enchiladas

Makes enough for: 6
Time required for proper preparation: 30 minutes
Suggested cooking time: 30 minutes
Total required: 1 hour

What to Use
- Water (3.5 c)
- Lime juice (1 T)
- Vegetable broth (.5 c low sodium, fat-free)
- Black beans (.6 c drained and rinsed)
- Tomato paste (1 T low-sodium)
- Kosher sea salt (as desired)
- Cumin (.5 tsp. ground)
- Mexican style crema (6 T)
- Onions (3 divided, sliced)
- Monterey Jack cheese (2 oz. shredded)
- Cheddar cheese (2.5 oz. shredded)
- Corn tortillas (12)
- Oregano (1 tsp.)
- Garlic (4 tsp. minced)
- Onion (2 c chopped)
- Coconut oil (2 tsp.)
- Enchilada sauce (28 oz. can red or green)

What to Do
- Preheat oven to 400F.
- Place a skillet on top of a stove over a burner set to medium heat. Place oil in the pan; swirl to coat. Add onion; cook until tender, stirring as needed
- Add garlic, oregano, cumin, and salt and let it cook for 2 minutes while still stirring before adding in the tomato paste and letting everything cook an additional minute.
- Add in the broth, beans, and beef and let everything cook another minute, still stirring. After you have removed it from heat, add in the lime juice.
- Wrap six tortillas at a time in a wet paper towel covering the top and the bottom. Microwave for 45 seconds or until soft. In each tortilla, at 3 T of the beef before rolling tightly.
- Add half a cup of the sauce to the bottom of a glass baking dish (13 x 9) that has been prepared using cooking spray before placing the enchiladas into the dish. Pour remaining enchilada sauce over the enchiladas. Top with the cheeses.
- Add the dish to the oven and let it bake at 400F for approximately 20 minutes. You are looking for it to be lightly browned and bubbly. Let the

enchiladas stand for 10 minutes. Top with the green onions and crema if serving immediately. This makes a great frozen dish.

Black Bean and Red Pepper Quinoa Salad

Makes enough for: 4
Time required for proper preparation: 10 minutes
Suggested cooking time: 15 minutes
Time total: 25 minutes

What to Use - Salad
- Quinoa (.75 c)
- Water (1.5 c)
- Salt (1 pinch)
- Green onion (.3 c thinly sliced)
- Red bell pepper (1 chopped)
- Cilantro (.5 c chopped)
- Black beans (1 can drained, rinsed)

What to Use - Dressing
- Lime juice (2 T)
- Seasoning salt (1 tsp.)
- Black pepper (as desired)
- Cumin (1 tsp. ground)
- Coconut oil (.25 c)
- Paprika or other chili powder (.5 tsp.)

What to Do
- Rinse the quinoa using a strainer before adding it, the salt and the water to a pot before placing it on the stove over a burner turned to high heat. Once it boils, turn the heat down and allow it to simmer while covered until all the water has been completely absorbed. Fluff the quinoa and set aside.
- Drain the beans into a colander in the sink and rinse with cold water until all the foam is gone. Drain beans until they are very dry (or pat with paper towels to speed it up.)
- Once the quinoa has cooled, add in the non-dressing ingredients and mix well. Portion it out into 8 containers and sprinkle some chopped cilantro on top. You can mix in the dressing right away or keep the dressing on the side and add in a little before eating. This meal will remain good for 3 days as long as it is refrigerated.

Asparagus and Farro Salad

Serves: 4
Time required for proper preparation: 20 minutes
Suggested cooking time: 30 minutes
Total required: 50 minutes

What to Use - Salad
- Farro (1 c)
- Asparagus (1 c sliced)
- Coconut oil (3 tsp.)
- Lemon juice (1 tsp.)
- Green onions (.6 c sliced)
- Parsley (.5 c chopped)
- Red pepper (1 diced)

What to Use - Dressing
- Capers (.3 c juice included)
- Sun-dried tomatoes (3 T chopped)
- Parsley (2 T chopped)
- Red wine vinegar (.3 c)
- Coconut oil (.3 c)
- Lemon juice (2 tsp.)
- Dijon mustard (1 tsp.)

What to Do
- Add the farro to a skillet before placing the skillet on the stove on top of a high/medium heat until it begins to brown. You will then want to turn off the heat before adding in 1.75 cups of boiling water to the skillet, as well as a pinch of salt. Turn the burner to low and let it cook for 20 minutes. Add a small amount of water if necessary.) Drain excess water.
- As the farro cooks, you will want to add the parsley, tomatoes, and capers to your food processor or blender and go nuts well. Add the pureed results into a bowl before adding in the red wine vinegar, Dijon and lemon juice before adding in the coconut oil and whisking well.
- After the farro has cooled, add it to a separate bowl and add .25 c of the previous bowl into this one.
- Add 2 tsp. coconut oil in a heavy pan, and sauté asparagus slices approximately 5 minutes or until done. Add in the remainder of the lemon juice and add the results to the bowl of farro
- Add the oil to the pan before placing it on top of a burner turned to a high/medium heat. Add in the red pepper and allow it to sauté for about 1 minute before adding it to the farro mixture and combining thoroughly.

- Add the chopped parsley and sliced green onions together in a bowl and mix well. Add dressing to your liking or keep on the side to add before serving. This will keep for 3 days in the fridge.

Black Bean Stew

Serves: 6
Time required for proper preparation: 15 minutes
Suggested cooking time: 75 minutes
Total required: 1 hour 30 minutes

What to Use
- Coconut oil (2 T)
- White onion (1 large diced)
- Black beans (7 c cooked, drained)
- Plum tomatoes (28 oz. diced)
- Cilantro stems (.25 c chopped, leaves reserved for serving)
- Kosher salt (2 tsp. more as needed)
- Scallion (1 sliced, for serving)
- Lime wedges (for serving)
- Diced avocado (for serving)

What to Do
- Place the oil in a heavy pot before placing the pot on the stove on top of a burner set to medium heat. Add onion and cook, stirring occasionally, until softened, 5 to 10 minutes. Add in the cilantro stems and cook an additional 5 minutes over high heat.
- Stir in beans, tomatoes and their juices, and the water. Let the results boil before reducing to medium.
- Cover the pot partially and simmer until tomatoes fall apart, between 1 hour and 1 hour 15 minutes. Top with avocado, scallion, cilantro leaves and lime wedges to serve.

Lentil Chili and Cornbread

Makes enough for: 6
Time required for proper preparation: 10 minutes
Suggested cooking time: 55 minutes
Total required: 65 minutes

What to Use
- Dry lentils (1.25 c)
- Coconut oil (2 T)
- Water (4 c)
- Onion (1 or 2 T minced)
- Vegetable broth (3 c)
- Tomatoes (15 oz. can)
- Garlic (1 clove minced)
- Chili powder (1.75 tsp.)
- Salt (.25 tsp.)
- Cayenne pepper (1 tsp.)
- Black pepper (as desired)
- Paprika (1 tsp.)

What to Do
- Prepare the lentils by rinsing them and sorting them before adding them to a pot along with the vegetable broth and water before placing the pot on the stove over a burner set to a high heat until it boils.
- Turn down the heat and let the pot simmer, covered, for half an hour.
- After the lentils have fully cooked, add in the rest of the ingredients and let everything simmer for 25 more minutes.

Garbanzo Bean Soup

Makes enough for: 8
Time required for proper preparation: 15 minutes
Suggested cooking time: 22 minutes
Total required: 37 minutes

What to Use
- Coconut oil
- Garlic (1 clove minced)
- Garbanzo beans (2 c cooked)
- Potato (1 diced)
- Vegetable broth (3 c)
- Salt (as desired)
- Pepper (as desired)
- Thyme (.3 tsp. dried)
- Carrot (1)
- Bay leaf (1)
- Onion (. 3 diced)
- Celery (1 stalk diced)

What to Do
- Start by sautéing the thyme, onion, celery, carrot and bay leaf on medium heat in a drizzle of oil.
- Wait 10 minutes before adding in the chickpeas, garlic, and potato and letting it all cook for 2 minutes.
- Mix in the broth before allowing it to simmer for 20 minutes and season as desired.
- At this point, you may choose to leave the soup chunky or make it smooth with an immersion or stand-up blender.

Herbed Balsamic Lentils with Polenta

Makes enough for: 4
Time required for proper preparation: 10 minutes
Suggested cooking time: 30 minutes
Total required: 40 minutes

What to Use
- Water (4 c)
- Onion (1 c diced)
- Carrots (2 c)
- Celery (1 c chopped)
- Garlic (4 T)
- Tomato paste (2 T)
- Oregano (.3 tsp. dried)
- Thyme (.3 tsp. dried)
- Brown lentils (.6c)
- Vegetable broth (5 c)
- Black pepper (1 tsp)
- Coconut oil (1 T)
- Salt (1 tsp.)
- Coconut oil (4 T)
- Cornmeal (.75 c)
- Pepper (1 tsp.)

What to Do
- Add the celery, onion, and carrots to a skillet set to a medium/high heat and let them sauté in Coconut oil for 2 minutes.
- After a few minutes, mix in the oregano, thyme, garlic and tomato paste.
- Cook the dry spices and garlic for another minute before adding the lentils.
- Heat them through, and then add the broth to the vegetable and lentil mixture. Cover and cook for 25 minutes.
- While the lentils are cooking, you'll prepare the polenta.
- Finish the lentils with balsamic vinegar and salt and pepper as desired. Serve over cheesy polenta.

Curried Lentils and Rice

Makes enough for: 6
Time required for proper preparation: 10 minutes
Suggested cooking time: 1 hour
Total required: 1 hour and 10 minutes

What to Use
- Vegetable broth (1 - 2 T)
- Granny Smith apple (1 diced)
- Onion (.3 chopped)
- Currants (.3 c)
- Curry powder (3 tsp.)
- Ginger (.3 tsp. ground)
- Vegetable bouillon cubes (3)
- Turmeric (.3 tsp.)
- Water (3.5 c)
- Lentils (.5 c dried)
- Brown rice (.75 c)

What to Do
- Add the broth to a soup pot before using it to sauté the 1 clove of garlic and the onion.
- Mix in the ginger, turmeric and curry powder and let everything cook for 2 minutes before adding in the rice and letting everything cook 2 minutes more, then adding in the rest of the ingredients except for the apples.
- Increase the heat until the pot boils before turning the heat back down and letting everything simmer for about half an hour. Add in the apples and simmer for another half an hour.
- Serve with a dollop of yogurt.

Japanese Red Bean Soup with Spinach Recipe

Makes enough for: 4
Time required for proper preparation: 15 minutes
Suggested cooking time: 35 minutes
Total required: 50 minutes

What to Use
- Red beans (.5 c soaked in water 4 hours or more)
- Bay leaf (1)
- Water (1.5 c)
- Onion (1 large, chopped)
- Carrots (2 cut into small slices)
- Celery (1 stalk cut into small slices)
- Shitake mushrooms (1 c cut into small slices)
- Coconut oil (1 T)
- Garlic (3 cloves cut into tiny pieces)
- Ginger (2 T grated)
- Vegetable stock (4 c)
- Sea salt (as desired)
- Thyme (1 tsp.)
- Cayenne pepper (as desired)
- Spinach (2 c chopped)
- Scallions (2 thinly sliced)

What to Do
- Remove the water from the beans. Place the beans, Kombu, bay leaf and water in a medium-sized pan. Bring water to a boil. Cover the pan and allow to simmer for approximately 1 hour or until just about tender.
- Turn the stove to low/medium, then in a large pot, add coconut oil. Mix in onions, carrots, celery, and sauté until soft and tender, for approximately 5 minutes.
- Add in the mushrooms, continue sautéing for approximately 5 minutes until mushrooms begin to soften and become golden.
- Mix in the ginger and garlic, cooking for about 1 minute.
- Without removing the liquid from the beans, add them in, as well as the stock, thyme, salt and cayenne as desired.
- Continue simmering for another 25 minutes, stirring every so often.
- When the beans and mushrooms are soft and tender, add in the spinach. Stir until the spinach has wilted
- Taste to adjust seasoning as desired.
- Serve the dish with the scallions as a garnish.

Sweet Potato Burgers

Up to 50 minutes prep, 30 minutes for setting, 8 minutes cook time. Makes about six servings.

Makes enough for: 6
Time required for proper preparation: 50 minutes
Suggested cooking time: 10 minutes
Total required: 60 minutes

What to Use
- Quinoa (1.5 c cooked)
- Black beans (1 15-oz. can drained, rinsed)
- Sweet potato (1 large peeled, cubed)
- Red onion (.5 c diced)
- Garlic (2 cloves minced)
- Cilantro (.5 c + 2 T chopped)
- Jalapeno (5 medium, diced, seed removed)
- Cumin (1 tsp. ground)
- Cajun seasoning (2 tsp.)
- Oat Flour (.25 c)
- Salt (as desired)
- Pepper (as desired)
- Coconut oil (2 T)
- Sprouts (as desired)
- Bib lettuce (6 leaves)
- Avocado (.5 large, diced)
- Plain Greek yogurt (.25 c)
- Lime juice (1 tsp.)
- Hot sauce (as desired)

What to Do
- Cook the sweet potatoes for about four minutes or until soft. If roasting the potatoes, place them on a baking tray in an oven pre-heated to 400F. Roast them for about 30 minutes. Remove the skins when cooked.
- Place the sweet potatoes into a blender. Add the black beans, Cajun seasoning, cumin, garlic, cilantro, and red onion and blend until smooth.
- In a large mixing bowl, transfer the blender ingredients in with the cooked quinoa. Stir together until combined. Season as desired
- Stir in the flour to thicken the mixture. You may not need the entire amount.
- Form the mixture into six "burgers," using about .5 c of the mixture for each patty. Place on parchment paper and cool them in the fridge for about 30 minutes.
- While cooling, make the avocado cream. In the blender or food processor, add the avocado, lime juice, and remaining cilantro. Pulse until creamy. Add to the fridge to cool with the patties.

- When ready to cook, warm coconut oil in a large skillet over high/medium heat. Place the "burgers" into the skillet and cook for about four minutes on each side. Serve with the cream on top when done.

Quesadilla and Avocado Salsa

Makes enough for: 4
Time required for proper preparation: 25 minutes
Suggested cooking time: 20 minutes
Total required: 45 minutes

What to Use
- Gluten-free tortillas (4)
- Monterey Jack cheese (1 c shredded)
- Baby spinach leaves (2 c lightly packed)
- Green chills (4 oz. diced)
- Avocado (1 smashed)
- Jalapeño peppers (1 or 2 seeded, halved)
- Lime juice (2 T)
- Coconut oil (2 T)
- Parmesan cheese (2 T)
- Garlic (1 clove)
- Salt (.5 tsp.)
- Cilantro (1 c)

What to Do
- Add all avocado sauce ingredients to a blender or food processor and blend until smooth.
- Place a skillet on top of the stove over a burner set to a medium heat before adding in a tortilla, 1 T green chilies, .25 c of cheese and. 5 c of spinach.
- Fold the results in half and let it cook for 2 minutes per side; repeat until all the ingredients have been used.
- Slice up the quesadillas and serve with the avocado sauce. They can be wrapped in foil and refrigerated for 3-4 days or frozen for 2-3 months. Reheat in a toaster oven for best results.

Poached Egg and Curry Potatoes

Makes enough for: 4
Time required for proper preparation: 10 minutes
Suggested cooking time: 30 minutes
Total required: 40 minutes

What to Use
- Potato, russet (2 large cubed)
- Ginger (1 in. nub peeled, minced)
- Garlic (2 cloves minced)
- Coconut oil (1 T)
- Curry powder (2 T)
- Tomato sauce (15 oz.)
- Eggs (4 large)
- Cilantro (.5 bunch chopped)

What to Do
- Warm water in a large stockpot and add the potatoes. Cover and boil on high heat for about five minutes. Drain and set aside.
- Warm the oil in a large skillet over low/medium heat. Add the garlic and ginger and cook for about two minutes. Stir in the curry powder and cook for another minute.
- Pour in the tomato sauce into the skillet and mix well. Increase the heat to medium and warm. Add salt if desired.
- Carefully add the potatoes, taking care not to splash the sauce. Mix to cover the potatoes. Add a bit of water to the skillet if the sauce is too thick.
- Push the sauce and potatoes aside, creating four wells to add the eggs. Crack each egg into the skillet. Cover and cook for about ten minutes or until eggs are well-cooked. Sprinkle cilantro on top, if desired.

Chapter 4: Seafood Recipes

Fish Sandwich

Makes enough for: 4
Time required for proper preparation: 10 minutes
Suggested cooking time: 10 minutes
Total required: 20 minutes

What to Use
- Salmon fillet (1 lb. quartered)
- Cajun seasoning (2 tsp.)
- Avocado (1 pitted, peeled)
- Mayonnaise (2 T)
- Wheat rolls (4)
- Arugula (1 c)
- Plum tomatoes (2 sliced thin)
- Red onion (.5 c sliced thin)
- Coconut oil (2 T)

What to Do
- Coat the grill in coconut oil before ensuring it is heated to high heat.
- Coat the fish using the seasoning before adding it to the grill and let it cook for approximately 3 minutes on each side.
- Mash the avocado before mixing it with the mayonnaise and spreading on the rolls prior to serving.
- Season as required, serve hot and enjoy.

Sardine Casserole

Makes enough for: 4
Time required for proper preparation: 15 minutes
Suggested cooking time: 40 minutes
Total required: 55 minutes

What to Use
- Bread crumbs (2 T)
- Basil (1 T)
- Garlic (2 cloves chopped)
- Cherry tomatoes (.5 lbs. diced)
- Sardines (17.5 oz.)
- Coconut oil (3 T)
- Russet potatoes (1 lb.)

What to Do
- Add the potatoes to a pot before covering them with salted water and letting the pot boil.
- Once it boils, turn the heat to low/medium before placing a lid on it and letting the potatoes cook for 20 minutes.
- Drain the potatoes and cover them in cold water to let them cool.
- Slice and peel the potatoes.
- Ensure your oven is heated to 350F.
- Add the coconut oil to a casserole dish and coat well.
- Alternate layers of potato and layers of sardine, adding the tomatoes to the sardine layers. Top with bread crumbs, basil, and garlic.
- Let the casserole cook for 20 minutes, serve hot and enjoy.

Mexican Salad with Mahi-Mahi

Makes enough for: 4
Time required for proper preparation: 75 minutes
Suggested cooking time: 20 minutes
Total required: 95 minutes

What to Use
- Ground beef (1 lb.)
- Pepper (as desired)
- Salt (as desired)
- Hot pepper sauce (as desired)
- Chili powder (.5 tsp.)
- Cumin (.5 T ground)
- Cilantro (.25 c chopped)
- Garlic (1 clove crushed)
- Agave sweetener (2 T)
- Lemon juice (1 T)
- Lime juice (2 T)
- Red wine vinegar (.5 c)
- Coconut oil (.5 c)
- Red onion (1 chopped)
- Corn kernels (10 oz. frozen)
- Red bell pepper (1 chopped)
- Green bell pepper (1 chopped)
- Cannellini beans (15 oz. rinsed, drained)
- Kidney beans (15 oz. rinsed, drained)
- Black beans (15 oz. drained, rinsed)
- Mahi-mahi (32 oz.)

What to Do
- In a serving bowl, combine the red onion, frozen corn, bell peppers, and beans and mix well.
- In a smaller separate bowl, combine the pepper, cumin, cilantro, hot pepper sauce, garlic, salt, sugar, lemon juice, lime juice, red wine vinegar and coconut oil and whisk well.
- Pour the dressing over the salad and toss well to coat; cover the salad with plastic wrap, and allow it to chill in the refrigerator and serve chilled.
- Prior to serving, season the fish as desired.
- Add the coconut oil to a pan before placing the pan on the stove over a burner set to medium heat.
- Add in the fish and let it cook for approximately 5 minutes on each side.

Flounder with Capers, Olives, and Tomatoes

This recipe needs 20 minutes to prepare, 20 minutes to cook and will make 4 servings.

Makes enough for: 4
Time required for proper preparation: 20 minutes
Suggested cooking time: 20 minutes
Total required: 40 minutes

What to Use
- Pepper (as desired)
- Extra virgin coconut oil (2 T)
- Basil (6 leaves torn)
- Flounder (1 lb. fillets)
- Parmesan cheese (3 T grated)
- Basil (6 leaves chopped)
- Lemon juice (1 tsp. fresh)
- Capers (.25 c)
- White wine (.25 c)
- Kalamata olives (24 chopped, pitted)
- Italian seasoning (1 pinch)
- Garlic (2 cloves chopped)
- Spanish onion (.5 chopped)
- Tomatoes (5 rinsed)

What to Do
- Ensure your oven is heated to 425F.
- Fill a saucepan with water and a pinch of salt before placing it on the stove on top of a burner that has been turned to high heat. Once the water boils, add in the tomatoes before pulling them right back out again. Ensure you have a bowl of cold water ready to add them to. Once they are cool enough to handle, remove the skin prior to chopping.
- Add the coconut oil to the skillet before placing the skillet on the stove on top of a burner set to medium heat. Add in the onion and let it cook for approximately 5 minutes until it is tender. Add in the Italian seasoning, garlic, and tomatoes and let everything cook for about 6 minutes.
- Add in half of the basil, the lemon juice, capers, wine, and olives before turning the heat down and mixing in the parmesan cheese. Let everything cook for approximately 15 minutes, and it has formed a thick sauce.
- Add the flounder to a baking dish before topping with sauce and basil leaves.
- Place the dish in the oven and let it cook for about 10 minutes until the flesh of the fish can easily be flaked with a fork.

Artichokes with Baked Cod

Makes enough for: 2
Time required for proper preparation: 20 minutes
Suggested cooking time: 15 minutes
Total required: 35 minutes

What to Use
- Red onion (.5 wedged)
- Zucchini (2 sliced)
- Garlic clove (1 minced)
- Thyme leaves (2 tsp.)
- Parsley (1 T chopped)
- Black pepper(as desired)
- Cod fillet (2, 6 oz.)
- Lemon juice (2 T)
- Lemon zest (2 T)
- Kalamata olives (8 pitted, chopped)
- Artichoke hearts (14 oz. can)
- Extra virgin coconut oil (1 T)

What to Do
- Ensure your oven has been heated to 450F.
- Coat a pan in the oil and place it on the stove above a burner that has been turned to a high/medium heat.
- Add the onions, thyme, garlic, and zucchini to the pan and let them sauté; you will be able to tell when they are finished because the onions will be practically see through.
- Remove the pan from the burner and mix in the zest, lemon juice, olives, and artichoke hearts.
- Season fish as desired before adding it to the pan and placing the pan in the oven for 15 minutes until the center of the fish is no longer see through.
- Top with parsley prior to serving.

Salmon Ceviche

Total preparation time (including cooking): 2 hours and 30 minutes
Yields: 3 servings

Makes enough for: 3
Time required for proper preparation: 120 minutes
Suggested cooking time: 10 minutes
Total required: 130 minutes

What to Use
- Salmon (5 oz.)
- Cilantro (1 T)
- Purple or yellow onion (.25 c)
- Black pepper (.25 tsp.)
- Fresh lemon juice (3 T)
- Coconut oil (2 T)

What to Do
- Chop the onion and the cilantro.
- Mix the cilantro, onion, black pepper and blend with the tuna.
- Mix in lemon juice.
- Cover and place in refrigerator to marinate for at least 2 hours.
- Add the coconut oil to a pan before placing the pan on the stove over a burner set to medium heat.
- Add in the fish and let it cook for approximately 5 minutes on each side

Tuna Salad

Makes enough for: 1
Time required for proper preparation: 10 minutes
Suggested cooking time: 0 minutes
Total required: 10 minutes

What to Use
- Pine nuts (2 T)
- Orange (1 segmented)
- Basil (2 T chopped)
- Wild Mushrooms (2.5 oz. sliced)
- Romaine lettuce (5 oz. torn)
- Extra virgin coconut oil (.5 T)
- Black pepper(as desired)
- Lemon juice (1 T +.5 tsp. lemon juice)
- Hummus (3 T)
- Green onion (1.5 oz. chopped)
- Celery (1.75 oz. chopped)
- Tuna (6 oz.)

What to Do
- Combine the pepper, the T of lemon juice, hummus, green onion, celery, and tuna together in a small bowl and stir together well.
- In a separate bowl, combine the remaining lemon juice and the extra virgin coconut oil before adding in half of the basil as well as the mushrooms and lettuce.
- Combine the two bowls and mix well before topping with the basil and the pine nuts.

Avocado and Tuna Lettuce Wrap

Makes enough for: 1
Time required for proper preparation: 5 minutes
Suggested cooking time: 0 minutes
Total required: 5 minutes

What to Use
- lettuce leaves (2 large)
- Tuna (8 oz.)
- Avocado (.5)
- Paleo mayo (2 T)
- Green olives (.25 c pitted, sliced)
- Pepper (as desired)
- Salt (as desired)
- Green chilies (2 T diced)

What to Do
- Chop the olives, scallion and green chilies before adding them to a mixing bowl. Mash the avocado before adding it in as well. The avocado should have a texture that appears creamy.
- Add in the mayonnaise as well as the tuna and mix well
- Add the results from the mixing bowl to the lettuce leaves, splitting the tuna in half.
- Roll like a burrito, serve and enjoy.

Tuna Panini

Makes enough for: 4
Time required for proper preparation: 10 minutes
Suggested cooking time: 15 minutes
Total required: 25 minutes

What to Use
- Coconut oil (2 tsp.)
- Salt (as desired)
- Black pepper (as desired)
- Wholegrain bread (8 slices)
- Lemon juice (1 tsp.)
- Capers (1 tsp. chopped)
- Kalamata olives (1 T chopped, pitted)
- Red onion (2 T minced)
- Artichoke hearts (2 T chopped)
- Feta cheese (.25 c crumbled)
- Plum tomato (1 chopped)
- Light tuna (12 oz. chunked)

What to Do
- Flake the tuna in a bowl with the help of a fork. Mix in the pepper, salt, lemon juice, capers, olives, onion, artichokes, feta, and tomato and combine well.
- Place.5 c of the tuna mixture on half of the slices. And top the sandwiches.
- Add the oil to a skillet and place the skillet on the stove over a burner set to a high/medium heat. Add 2 panini to the skillet at a time, and cook the first side for 2 minutes; turn the heat down to low/medium and cook the other side for 2 minutes.
- Add additional oil for the second set of sandwiches as needed.

Sweet Potatoes, Tuna, and Capers

Makes enough for: 2
Time required for proper preparation: 10 minutes
Suggested cooking time: 30 minutes
Total required: 40 minutes

What to Use
- Salt (as desired)
- Pepper (as desired)
- Capers (1 T)
- Green onion (1 cut into rings)
- Greek yogurt (2 T)
- Coconut oil (.5 T)
- Chili powder (1 T)
- Tuna (8 oz.)
- Sweet Potatoes (4)

What to Do
- Ensure your air fryer is set to 320F.
- Soak the potatoes for half an hour before drying them and covering them using the coconut oil.
- Place them in the basket, place the basket in the air fryer and let the potatoes cook for 30 minutes.
- While the potatoes are cooking, combine the chili powder, yogurt, and tuna in a bowl before adding pepper, salt and half of the ringed green onion.
- Slice the potatoes in half and hallow them out enough to add in the tuna mixture, capers, and the remaining green onion.

Yellow Fin Tuna with Poke

Makes enough for: 2
Time required for proper preparation: 5 minutes
Suggested cooking time: 10 minutes
Total required: 15 minutes

What to Use
- Salt (as desired)
- Pepper (as desired)
- Red grapefruit (.25)
- Pili nuts (.25 c)
- Sesame seeds (1 T)
- Sesame oil (2 T)
- Avocado (.5)
- Cilantro (5 sprigs)
- Coconut aminos (1 T)
- Tuna (8 oz. grilled)

What to Do
- Slice the tuna into.25 in. cubes and add to a large mixing bowl before mixing in the salt, pepper, sesame oil and coconut aminos and toss gently.
- Add in the grapefruit, pili nuts, avocado, and cilantro and mix well.
- Divide the results into two bowls and top with sesame seeds prior to serving.

Cheesy Tuna Casserole

Makes enough for: 4
Time required for proper preparation: 10 minutes
Suggested cooking time: 15 minutes
Total required: 25 minutes

What to Use
- Tuna (two 6-oz. cans, drained)
- Green beans (16-oz. bag, French-cut, frozen)
- Mushrooms (3 oz., fresh, sliced)
- Coconut oil (2 T)
- Chicken broth (.5 c)
- Heavy cream (.75 c)
- Onion (2 T chopped fine)
- Salt and pepper (as desired)
- Xanthan gum (optional)
- Celery (1 stalk, hashed fine)
- Cheddar cheese (4-8 oz., shredded)

What to Do
- Cook the green beans in a medium pot. Drain well.
- Place the coconut oil, celery, mushrooms, and onion in a pan and place the pan on top of the stove over a burner turned to medium heat and let everything cook for approximately 5 minutes or until done.
- Add the broth. Boil, letting the liquid cook down by half.
- Stir in the cream. Let come back up to a boil.
- Turn down the heat until the sauce is thickened, stirring frequently. Don't let it boil over.
- Season as desired.
- Put the mushroom mixture and tuna into the green beans.
- Add salt and pepper if needed.
- Put the cheese in it, thoroughly mixing it in.
- Put the mixture into a 1.5 or 2-quart casserole dish.
- Microwave or bake until hot.

Caper Salad with a Mediterranean Twist

Makes enough for: 4
Time required for proper preparation: 10 minutes
Suggested cooking time: 0 minutes
Total required: 10 minutes

What to Use

- Tomatoes (2 large)
- Pepper (as desired)
- Salt (as desired)
- Lemon juice (1 T)
- Capers (1 T)
- Basil (2 T)
- Red peppers (2 T roasted, chopped)
- Red onion (2 T minced)
- Kalamata olives (.25 c chopped)
- Mayonnaise (.25 c)
- Tuna (10 oz.)

What to Do

- In a large bowl, mix everything, save the tomatoes together.
- Cut the tops of the tomatoes off, remove the insides, add the tuna mixture to the tomatoes, serve and enjoy.

Fish Soup

Makes enough for: 6
Time required for proper preparation: 15 minutes
Suggested cooking time: 4 hours and 20 minutes
Total required: 4 hours and 35 minutes

What to Use
- Cod (1 lb. cubed)
- Shrimp (1 lb. deveined, peeled)
- Salt and pepper (as desired)
- Fennel seed (.25 tsp. crushed)
- Basil (1 tsp.)
- Bay leaves (2)
- Dry white wine (.5 c)
- Orange juice (.5 c)
- Black olives (.25 c sliced)
- Mushrooms (2.5 oz.)
- Tomato sauce (8 oz.)
- Chicken broth (28 oz.)
- Tomatoes (14.5 oz. can diced, drained)
- Garlic (2 cloves minced)
- Bell pepper (.5 chopped)
- Onion (1 chopped)

What to Do
- Add the pepper, fennel, basil, bay, wine, juice, olives, mushroom, tomato sauce, chicken broth, tomatoes, garlic, bell pepper, and onion into a crockpot, cover it and let everything cook at a low temperature for 4 hours.
- Add in the cod as well as the shrimp, return the lid to the crockpot and let it cook until the shrimp turn opaque, which should take 20 minutes.
- Serve hot and enjoy.

Fish Cakes

Makes enough for: 4
Time required for proper preparation: 2 hours and 30 minutes
Suggested cooking time: 10 minutes
Total required: 2 hours and 40 minutes

What to Use
- Whole wheat flour (4 T)
- Shrimp (6.5 oz.)
- Tuna (9 oz.)
- Bread crumbs (.5 c)
- Italian seasoning (1 T)
- Chili peppers (2 seeded)
- Basil (6 leaves)
- Egg (1)
- Sun-dried tomatoes (5 chopped)
- Garlic (4 cloves)
- Onion (.5)
- Scallops (6 oz.)
- Coconut oil (4 T)

What to Do
- Coat a pan in 1 T oil and place it on the stove above a burner that has been turned to a high/medium heat.
- Add in the scallops and let them cook until they are completely white.
- In a food processor, mix in 1 T coconut oil, the egg, tomatoes, garlic, and onion before adding in the seasoning, chilies, basil and parsley and process on the medium setting.
- Add in the shrimp, scallops and tuna and process on a low setting.
- Add in the breadcrumbs and keep processing until everything binds together.
- Make the results into patties before adding them to a plate and placing the plate in the refrigerator for at least 2 hours.
- Coat a pan in the remaining oil and place it on the stove above a burner that has been turned to medium heat.
- Cook the patties in the pan until both sides have turned a golden brown.

Cod with Roasted String Beans

Makes enough for: 3
Time required for proper preparation: 10 minutes
Suggested cooking time: 10 minutes
Total required: 20 minutes

What to Use
- Horseradish (as desired)
- Red onion (.5 wedged)
- Black pepper(as desired)
- Red pepper flakes (as desired)
- Dill (3 T chopped)
- Garlic (2 cloves minced)
- Lemon zest (2 T)
- Lemon juice (2 T)
- Extra virgin coconut oil (2 T)
- Codd (16 oz.)

What to Do
- Ensure your oven is heated to 450F.
- Mix the pepper, red pepper flakes, 2 T dill, garlic, lemon zest, lemon juice, and extra virgin coconut oil together in a bowl and combine well. Use half of the results to coat the fish.
- Add the onion and string beans to the remaining oil mixture before spreading the vegetables onto a baking sheet.
- Add the vegetables to the oven and let them cook for 15 minutes before adding the cod to the top of the vegetables face down.
- Let the fish cook for 12 minutes or until the fish looks opaque in its center.
- Season as desired.

Shrimp and Chicken Jambalaya

Makes enough for: 8
Time required for proper preparation: 15 minutes
Suggested cooking time: 6 hours
Total required: 6 hours and 15 minutes

What to Use
- Parsley (2 T)
- Hot sauce (1 T)
- Shrimp (1 lb. peeled, deveined)
- Long grain rice (7 oz.)
- Chicken broth (14 oz. can)
- Tomatoes (14.5 oz. can diced)
- Paprika (.25 tsp)
- Thyme (.5 tsp.)
- Cajun Seasoning (2 tsp.)
- Turkey kielbasa (4 oz. 25-inch slices)
- Garlic (2 cloves minced)
- Celery (1 c chopped)
- Green Bell Pepper (1 c chopped)
- Onion (2 c chopped)
- Chicken thighs (.75 lb. skinless, boneless, 1-inch pieces)
- Chicken breasts (1 lb. skinless, boneless, 1-inch pieces)
- Coconut oil (1 T)

What to Do
- On high heat, preheat a large skillet with a bit of oil. Cook the chicken for about 5 minutes, then place it in the slow cooker.
- Mix the garlic, celery, bell pepper and onion in the skillet before sautéing for 4 minutes. Add the results plus the kielbasa,
- Put this mixture with Cajun seasoning, thyme, paprika, tomatoes, chicken broth, and the turkey kielbasa. Cook on for 6 hours.
- Prepare your rice to your preference, then add the cooked rice and remaining ingredients to the slow cooker. Cook on high for an additional 15 minutes. Garnish with the parsley, and enjoy!

Halibut with Mango and Ginger Salsa

Makes enough for: 2
Time required for proper preparation: 15 minutes
Suggested cooking time: 10 minutes
Total required: 25 minutes

What to Use
- Coconut oil (2 T)
- Halibut (1 lb.)
- Mango (1 diced, peeled)
- Red onion (1 chopped)
- Ginger (1 tsp. grated)
- Garlic (2 cloves minced)
- Red pepper (1 chopped)
- Lime (1 juiced)
- Cilantro (.5 bunches)

What to Do
- Season the fish as desired.
- Add the coconut oil to a pan before placing the pan on the stove over a burner set to medium heat.
- Add in the fish and let it cook for approximately 5 minutes on each side.
- Combine the remaining ingredients and add them to the top of the fish, serve hot and enjoy.

Salmon with Roasted Cauliflower

Makes enough for: 2
Time required for proper preparation: 10 minutes
Suggested cooking time: 10 minutes
Total required: 20 minutes

What to Use
- Lemon (.5 wedged)
- Black pepper(as desired)
- Cayenne pepper (1 tsp.)
- Dill (3 T chopped)
- Garlic (2 cloves minced)
- Lemon zest (2 T)
- Lemon juice (2 T)
- Extra virgin coconut oil (2 T)

What to Do
- Ensure your oven is heated to 450F.
- Mix the pepper, red pepper flakes, 2 T dill, garlic, lemon zest, lemon juice, and extra virgin coconut oil together in a bowl and combine well. Use half of the results to coat the fish.
- Add the lemon and cauliflower to the remaining oil mixture before spreading the vegetables onto a baking sheet.
- Add the vegetables to the oven and let them cook for 15 minutes before adding the salmon to the top of the vegetables face down.
- Let the fish cook for 12 minutes or until the fish looks opaque in its center.
- Season as desired.

Crab Salad Cakes

Makes enough for: 4
Time required for proper preparation: 10 minutes
Suggested cooking time: 5 minutes
Total required: 15 minutes

What to Use
- Black pepper (.5 tsp.)
- Salt (.5 tsp.)
- Extra virgin coconut oil (1 T)
- Swiss cheese (.5 c shredded)
- Hot sauce (2 dashes)
- Old Bay seasoning (.25 tsp.)
- Mayonnaise (1 T)
- Lemon juice (4 tsp.)
- Scallion (1 chopped)
- Red bell pepper (.25 c chopped)
- Celery (.3 c chopped)
- Crab meat (8 oz.)
- asparagus spears (4 sliced)

What to Do
- Pace the rack high in the oven and heat your broiler.
- Microwave the asparagus in a covered bowl with 1 tsp. water for 30 seconds.
- Mix in the seasonings as desired as well as the mayonnaise, lemon juice, scallion, bell pepper, celery, and crab.
- For the results into 4 patties and top with the cheese.
- Broil the patties for 3 minutes.

Salmon with Kale

Makes enough for: 4
Time required for proper preparation: 20 minutes
Suggested cooking time: 13 minutes
Total required: 33 minutes

What to Use
- Black pepper (.5 tsp.)
- Salt (.5 tsp.)
- Extra virgin coconut oil (1 T)
- Lemon wedges (4)
- Dill (1 T chopped, fresh)
- Horseradish (2 tsp.)
- Sour cream (.25 c)
- Salmon (1 lb.)
- Kale (1 lb., chopped, stems removed)
- Water (.25 c)
- Chicken broth (1 c)
- Shallot (1 sliced thin)

What to Do
- Add the oil to a pan before placing the pan on the stove over a burner set to medium heat. Mix in .5 lbs. of kale, the water, and the broth before letting the kale wilt for 60 seconds. Mix in the rest of the kale and let it cook for 8 minutes.
- Season the fish as desired before placing it atop the kale, cover the pan and let the fish cook approximately 5 minutes or until done.
- While the fish cooks, in a small bowl, mix together the dill, horseradish and sour cream.
- Top the fish with the results and garnish with the lemon.

Coconut Amino Infused Salmon

Makes enough for: 4
Time required for proper preparation: 10 minutes
Suggested cooking time: 12 minutes
Total required: 22 minutes

What to Use
- Coconut aminos (1.5 c)
- Sesame oil (1 T toasted)
- Coconut oil (1 T)
- Green onions (3 chopped)
- Garlic (3 cloves)
- Salmon filet (4)
- Green beans (.75 lbs.)
- Mushrooms (1 lb.)
- Bell peppers (3 sliced thin, seeds removed)

What to Do
- Ensure your oven has been heated to 450F.
- Add a baking pan to the oven for the salmon as well as two for use with the vegetables.
- Add the garlic, oil, green onions, and coconut aminos to your food processor or blender and go nuts for 30 seconds.
- Coat the salmon using the results.
- In a mixing bowl, and the peppers, mushrooms and green beans and combine thoroughly before adding the remaining sauce and coating well.
- Add the items to their respective pans and let them bake for 12 minutes.

Orange Roughy Fillet

Makes enough for: 2
Time required for proper preparation: 5 minutes
Suggested cooking time: 12 minutes
Total required: 17 minutes

What to Use
- Italian seasoned bread crumbs (2 T)
- Worcestershire sauce (1 tsp.)
- Lemon juice (1.5 tsp.)
- Dijon mustard (1 T)
- Orange roughy (8 oz.)

What to Do
- Start by making sure your oven is heated to 450F.
- Prepare a baking dish (11 x 7) by spraying it with cooking spray before adding in the fish.
- In a small bowl, combine the Worcestershire sauce, lemon juice, and mustard and mix well. Spread the results over the filet evenly before coating in breadcrumbs.
- Place the baking dish in the oven for approximately 12 minutes; you will know the fish is ready when it flakes easily when pressed with a fork.
- Slice in half prior to serving and serve hot.

Baked Shrimp

Makes enough for: 4
Time required for proper preparation: 5 minutes
Suggested cooking time: 10 minutes
Total required: 15 minutes

What to Use
- Shrimp (1 lb. peeled, deveined)
- Low-sodium soy sauce (2 tsp.)
- Olive oil (1 tsp.)
- Creole seasoning (2 tsp.)
- Parsley (2 tsp. dried)
- Honey (1 T)
- Lemon juice (2 T)

What to Do
- Start by making sure your oven is heated to 450F.
- Prepare a baking dish (11 x 7) by spraying it with cooking spray.
- Add in the soy sauce, olive oil, Creole seasoning, dried parsley, and honey and combine thoroughly. Add in the shrimp and toss to coat.
- Place the baking dish in the oven for 8 minutes, stirring every 2 minutes. The shrimp should be a light pink color when ready to serve.

Chapter 5: Poultry Recipes

Chicken Cacciatore with Spaghetti Squash

Makes enough for: 6
Time required for proper preparation: 60 minutes
Suggested cooking time: 30 minutes
Total required: 90 minutes

What to Use
- Chicken thighs (4 boneless, skinless, bite-size)
- Onion (1 medium, diced)
- Bell peppers (1 large, bite-size)
- Garlic (2 cloves, minced)
- Dried thyme (.5 tsp)
- Chicken stock (1 cup)
- Diced tomatoes (one 28-ounce can)
- Tomato sauce (one 8-ounce can)
- Dried basil (.5 tsp.)
- Salt (as desired)
- Pepper (as desired)
- Yellow squash (.5, diced)
- Dried oregano (.5 tsp)
- Spaghetti squash (1, small)

What to Do
- Dice the veggies. Set them aside.
- Cut the chicken up. Season it as desired.
- Place the chicken in a Dutch oven and let it brown for about 8 minutes.
- Add in the onion, garlic and bell pepper and let them cook for approximately 5 minutes or until the onions soften.
- Add the chicken tomato sauce, tomatoes, and the chicken stock.
- Season as desired and mix well before letting everything boil.
- Turn the heat to low and let everything cook for 30 minutes.
- Add the yellow squash. Cook between 15 and 30 more minutes.

Celery Fries and Chicken

Makes enough for: 6
Time required for proper preparation: 15 minutes
Suggested cooking time: 20 minutes
Total required: 35 minutes

What to Use - *Chicken*
- Coconut oil (2 T)
- Salt (as needed)
- Chicken breasts (4)
- Pepper (as needed)

What to Use - *Celery Fries*
- Salt (.5 tsp)
- Pepper (.25 tsp)
- Root celery (1.5 lbs.)
- Coconut oil (2 T)

What to Do
- Ensure your oven is on and turn to 400F.
- Cube the chicken before adding it to a large mixing bowl before adding in 2 T coconut oil and seasoning as needed. Allow the chicken to marinate for at least 15 minutes.
- At the same time, cut the root celery into strips and place it in a large bowl before adding in the remaining coconut oil and seasoning as needed. Shake well to coat.
- Place the celery strips and chicken on a baking sheet before placing the sheet in the oven to bake for 20 minutes.

Chicken Thighs with Turmeric and Cumin

Makes enough for: 2
Time required for proper preparation: 5 minutes
Suggested cooking time: 15 minutes
Total required: 20 minutes

What to Use
- Black pepper (as desired)
- Water (.5 c)
- Hot sauce (1 T)
- Black molasses (1 T)
- Honey (.25 c)
- Coconut oil (2 T)
- Lemon juice (.5 T)
- Turmeric (.5 tsp.)
- Ginger (.5 tsp.)
- Coriander (.5 tsp.)
- Cumin (.5 tsp.)
- Chicken thighs (1 lb.)

What to Do
- Combine the spices in a small bowl and mix well. Use the results to coat the chicken thoroughly before placing it in the Instant Pot cooker pot along with the coconut oil and choose the sauté option, leaving the cooker uncovered. Brown the chicken thighs evenly.
- Remove the chicken from the pot before adding in a little water, be prepared for it to boil quickly. Once the noise dies down, remove the brown bits from the bottom of the Instant Pot cooker pot before returning the chicken to the pot and setting the pressure to high and the time to 15 minutes.
- While the chicken is cooking, combine the lemon, molasses, and honey together in a small bowl.
- Once the timer goes off, select the instant pressure release option and remove the lid.
- Remove the chicken and cover it with foil to keep warm. Turn the Instant Pot cooker back to sauté before adding the honey mixture to the pot and letting everything boil, whisking regularly until the sauce thickens.
- Dip each chicken thigh into the sauce prior to serving.

Chicken Cheese Steak

Makes enough for: 5
Time required for proper preparation: 20 minutes
Suggested cooking time: 5 hours
Total required: 5 hours and 20 minutes

What to Use
- Black pepper (as desired)
- Sea salt (as desired)
- Oopsie Bread (6 slices)
- Steak seasoning (2 T)
- Garlic cloves (2 chopped)
- Provolone cheese (6 slices)
- Green peppers (2 sliced thin)
- Onion (1 sliced)
- Light Coconut oil (2 T)
- Chicken breasts (1 lb.)

What to Do
- Thinly slice the chicken into strips before adding it to a bowl and seasoning with steak seasoning, pepper, and salt as needed.
- Add the coconut oil to the slow cooker before adding in the green peppers as well as the onions, and then top it all with the chicken.
- Cover the slow cooker and let it cook on low heat for 5 hours.
- Divide the results into 6 servings and add the results to each roll before topping with the cheese and toasting for 2 minutes prior to serving.

Chicken Korma

Makes enough for: 3
Time required for proper preparation: 15 minutes
Suggested cooking time: 30 minutes
Total required: 35 minutes

What to Use
- Chicken breast (16 oz. grilled)
- Cooking cream (100 milliliters 35 percent fat)
- Coconut oil (5 T)
- Cinnamon (1 stick)
- Curry (.5 T)
- Garlic (2 cloves chopped)
- Ginger (2 T grated)
- Cardamom (7 pods)
- Bay (2 leaves)
- Onion (1)
- Cayenne pepper (as desired)
- Coconut milk (30 grams)
- Salt (.5 tsp.)
- Water (3 T)

What to Do
- Cut the onion so that one half is chopped and the other is thinly sliced.
- Place the coconut milk and coconut oil together into a frying pan before adding a medium heat.
- Once the mixture is heated, add in the cardamom pods, bay leaves, and cinnamon sticks and let them sizzle for just a few seconds.
- Add the onion slices into the mixture and allow them to become a light brown.
- Mix the salt, curry, cayenne pepper, garlic, ginger, and chopped onion together well before adding in the cooking cream.
- Add the results to the chicken and mix well.
- Add the water to the pan before letting it simmer for 10 minutes.

Teriyaki Chicken

Makes enough for: 2
Time required for proper preparation: 2 hours and 15 minutes
Suggested cooking time: 25 minutes
Total required: 2 hours and 40 minutes

What to Use
- Black pepper (as needed)
- Salt (as needed)
- Chicken breast (1.5 lbs.)
- Coconut oil (3 T)
- Sweetener (as desired)
- Powdered ginger (1 T)
- Powdered garlic (1 T)
- White vinegar (1 T)
- Worcestershire sauce (1 T)
- Soy sauce (.5 c)

What to Do
- Combine the Worcestershire sauce, coconut oil, sweetener, soy sauce, pepper, salt, ginger, garlic, and vinegar together using a large bowl.
- Add in the chicken, cover the bowl and let the chicken marinate for 2 hours.
- Add the chicken to a frying pan before placing the pan on the stove over a burner turned to a medium heat.
- Cook the chicken until the marinade has nearly completely evaporated, and the internal temperature has reached 165 degrees F.

Lemon Chicken

Makes enough for: 3
Time required for proper preparation: 2 hours and 15 minutes
Suggested cooking time: 15 minutes
Total required: 2 hours and 30 minutes

What to Use
- Salt (as desired)
- Pepper (1 tsp.)
- Chicken breast (500 grams)
- Lemon juice (1 T)
- Rosemary (1 T ground)
- Coconut oil (.75 c)
- Olives (15)
- Camembert (50 grams)

What to Do
- Begin by mixing together the pepper, rosemary, coconut oil and lemon juice to make the marinade for the chicken.
- Add the chicken and let it marinate for 2 hours. After it has finished marinating, add salt if you prefer.
- Top the chicken with olives and the camembert prior to serving.
- Place the chicken in a glass baking pan and then place it in the oven for about 15 minutes or until the chicken hits 165F internally.

Zucchini with Feta and Chicken

Makes enough for: 2
Time required for proper preparation: 15 minutes
Suggested cooking time: 20 minutes
Total required: 35 minutes

What to Use
- Salt (as desired)
- Pepper (as desired)
- Chicken breast (500 grams)
- Rosemary (1 T)
- Coconut oil (4 T)
- Lemon Juice (2 T)
- Feta cheese (50 grams)
- Zucchini (2)

What to Do
- Ensure your oven is preheated to 375F
- Prepare the feta cheese, zucchini, and chicken breast by cutting it into cubes.
- Add 1 T of the olive oil into a frying pan and heat it on a high/medium heat before sautéing the zucchini for around 6 minutes.
- Mix together the rest of the oil with the pepper, salt, and rosemary before placing the chicken onto a cooking tray and covering it with the oil mixture.
- Add the feta cheese and zucchini cubes once the chicken has been coated.
- Place tinfoil over the top of the tray, taking special care to leave room in the tinfoil for the steam to escape.
- Bake for 25 minutes.

Off the Cobb Salad

Makes enough for: 1
Time required for proper preparation: 10 minutes
Suggested cooking time: 0 minutes
Total required: 10 minutes

What to Use
- Spinach (1 c)
- Egg (1, hard-boiled)
- Bacon (2 strips)
- Chicken breast (2 oz. grilled)
- Campari tomato (one half of tomato)
- Avocado (one fourth, sliced)
- White vinegar (half of a tsp.)
- Coconut oil (1 T)

What to Do
- Cook the bacon completely and cut or slice into small pieces.
- Chop remaining ingredients into bite-size pieces.
- Place all ingredients, including chicken and bacon, in a bowl, toss ingredients in oil and vinegar.
- Enjoy!

Chicken Casserole

Makes enough for: 4
Time required for proper preparation: 35 minutes
Suggested cooking time: 10 minutes
Total required: 45 minutes

What to Use
- Grass-fed Coconut oil (2 T)
- Salt (as needed)
- Pepper (as needed)
- Heavy whipping cream (1.3 c)
- Separated chicken breast (1.5 lbs.)
- Pitted olives (.5 c)
- Green pesto (4 oz)
- Feta cheese (.5 lbs. shredded)
- Garlic clove (1 chopped)

What to Do
- Ensure your oven is on and turned to 400F.
- Mix together the pesto and the heavy cream in a mixing bowl.
- Add the cheese, chicken, olives, and garlic to a baking dish and cover with the peso/cream mixture.
- Add the dish to the oven and let it cook for 30 minutes.

BLT Chicken Salad

Makes enough for: 1
Time required for proper preparation: 15 minutes
Suggested cooking time: 0 minutes
Total required: 15 minutes

What to Use
- Boneless chicken breast (1, grilled)
- Leaf lettuce (2 c, chopped)
- Tomato (.5 small)
- Swiss cheese (.5-oz., julienned)
- Bacon (1-2 strips, crisp and crumbled)
- Egg (.5 hard-boiled, sliced in half)
- Ranch dressing (2 T)
- Black pepper (dash)
- Parsley (pinch, fresh, chopped, optional)
- Sliced cucumber (chopped, optional)
- Chives (chopped, optional)
- Green peppers (slivered, optional)
- Avocado (chopped, optional)
- Sunflower seeds (optional)

What to Do
- Add the sliced chicken to a large plate covered in lettuce.
- Top the chicken with the remaining ingredients.

California Grilled Chicken Avocado-Mango Salad

Makes enough for: 4
Time required for proper preparation: 15 minutes
Suggested cooking time: 0 minutes
Total required: 15 minutes

What to Use
- Chicken breast (12-oz. breast, grilled, sliced)
- Avocado (1 c, diced)
- Mango (1 c, diced from 1.5 mangos)
- Red onion (2 T)
- Red Coconut oil lettuce (6 c)

What to Use - Vinaigrette
- Balsamic vinegar (2 T white)
- Salt (as desired)
- Pepper (as desired)
- Coconut oil (2 T)

What to Do
- Whisk all vinaigrette ingredients together. Set aside.
- Fill 4 salad plates with baby greens.
- Toss the onion, mango, avocado, and chicken together.
- Plate the chicken atop the baby greens and top with vinaigrette prior to serving.

Chicken Curry

Makes enough for: 6
Time required for proper preparation: 30 minutes
Suggested cooking time: 40 minutes
Total required: 70 minutes

What to Use

- Chicken breasts (1.5 breasts)
- Cauliflower (1 head)
- Onion powder (.5 tsp.)
- Thai Kitchen Lite Coconut Milk (1 can)
- Hot curry powder (2 T)
- Garam masala (1 T)
- Coconut oil (.5 T)
- Green beans (2 c, frozen)
- Garlic powder (.5 tsp)
- Salt (as desired)
- Pepper (as desired)

What to Do

- Cut up the chicken into chunks.
- Coat the chicken chunks in half curry powder and half garam masala.
- Take the chicken out and put it into a deep pot. Leave the burned pieces and coconut oil in the frying pan because they are flavorful.
- Add coconut milk to the frying pan and scratch off all of the burned bits.
- Pour the coconut milk and the burned bits over the chicken that is in the deep pot.
- Add the remaining spices.
- Boil on a low/medium heat for half an hour.
- Add green beans. Continue cooking, uncovered to let the sauce thicken.
- Meanwhile, boil the cauliflower in water and 1 T of coconut oil in a separate pot.
- Mash the cauliflower until it is in small pieces. Season as needed.

Spaghetti Squash Chicken Alfredo

Makes enough for: 4
Time required for proper preparation: 15 minutes
Suggested cooking time: 20 minutes
Total required: 35 minutes

What to Use - Meal
- Garlic powder (1 tsp.)
- Sea salt (.5 tsp.)
- Basil for garnish
- Medium spaghetti squash (1)
- Chicken breast(1 lb.)
- Coconut oil (2 T)
- Juice of half a lemon

What to Use - Sauce
- Bone broth (.25 c)
- Medium cauliflower chopped (1)
- Coconut milk (.25 c)
- Coconut oil (1 T)
- Garlic powder (1 tsp.)
- Sea salt (.5 tsp.)

What to Do
- Preheat the oven to 400F
- Slice the squash in half and spoon out the seeds. Bake in the oven for 45-50 minutes or until the strands easily pull.
- Season the chicken breast with lemon, salt, and garlic and allow to marinate for about an hour in the fridge.
- Heat cooking fat of choice over medium heat and add the chicken.
- Add the cauliflower to a medium pot and fill about 60 percent of the way with water.
- Heat the cauliflower on medium heat and bring to a low simmer for about 8-10 minutes or until cauliflower is soft.
- Strain the cauliflower and allow it to cool.
- Add the cooled cauliflower to a high-speed blender with the remainder of the ingredients and blend until smooth.
- Either scoop the squash out of the shell or keep it in.
- Add the sauce and combine, reserving some to add over the top.
- Add the sliced chicken, some extra sauce, and basil for garnish.
- Serve and enjoy!

Low-Carb Pizza

Makes enough for: 2
Time required for proper preparation: 15 minutes
Suggested cooking time: 30 minutes
Total required: 45 minutes

What to Use
- Salt (.5 tsp.)
- Egg (1 large)
- White wine vinegar (1 tsp.)
- Cream cheese (2 T)
- Almond flour (.75 c)
- Mozzarella cheese (2 c divided, shredded)
- Grilled chicken (.5 lb.)
- Coconut oil (1 T grass fed)
- Oregano (.5 tsp. dried)
- Tomato sauce (.5 c unsweetened)

What to Do
- Start by making sure your oven is heated to 400F.
- Add the cream cheese and mozzarella cheese to a small pan before placing this pan on the stove on top of a burner set to medium heat.
- Stir to mix and continue stirring until both kinds of cheese have melted. Add in the .5 tsp. salt, the egg, and 1 tsp. white wine vinegar and mix thoroughly.
- Coat your hands in oil before taking the dough and flattening it out onto parchment paper so that it ends up being roughly 8 inches around. A rolling pin will also work if available.
- Using a fork, create a number of holes in the dough to prevent it from rising before placing it on a baking sheet and letting it bake for approximately 11 minutes.
- Add the toppings to the pizza, starting with the sauce, before placing it on a baking sheet and baking for 15 minutes.
- Top with oregano prior to serving.

Chapter 6: Beef Recipes

Fajita and Poblano Kabobs

Makes enough for: 3
Time required for proper preparation: 60 minutes
Suggested cooking time: 20 minutes
Total required: 80 minutes

What to Use - Marinade
- Black pepper (as needed)
- Salt (as needed)
- Flank steak (1 lb. sliced thin)
- Red pepper flakes (.25 tsp.)
- Sweet paprika (.25 tsp.)
- Oregano (.25 tsp.)
- Garlic powder (.25 tsp.)
- Lime juice (.5 T)
- Coconut aminos (.25 cups)

What to Use - Kabobs
- Red onion (.5 chopped)
- Red bell pepper (1 chopped)
- Yellow bell pepper (1 chopped)

What to Use - Poblano Pesto
- Coconut oil (2 T)
- Lime juice (.5 T)
- Cilantro (.5 cups)
- Poblano pepper (1 roasted)

What to Do
- Place the marinade ingredients as well as the steak into a dish with a lid and ensure the meat is well coated. Let the marinade chill for at least 2 hours.
- Skewer the meat and vegetables as desired before heating a grill pan in the oil and place it on the stove above a burner that has been turned to medium heat. Brush each kabob with the marinade before cooking each side for approximately 4 minutes.
- As the kabobs are cooking, add the pesto ingredients to a blender and blend well.
- Add the pesto to the kabobs prior to serving.

Steak Salad

Makes enough for: 4
Time required for proper preparation: 15 minutes
Suggested cooking time: 0 minutes
Total required: 15 minutes

What to Use
- Pepper (as desired)
- Salt (as desired)
- Carrots (3 sliced)
- Red leaf lettuce (1 head torn)
- Dijon mustard (1 T)
- Coconut oil (2 T)
- Radishes (8 quartered)
- Garlic (1 clove minced)
- White wine vinegar (2 T)
- Snap peas (8 oz. halved, steamed)
- Skirt steak (1 lb. halved)

What to Do
- Heat your broiler before placing the steak on top of a baking sheet lined with tinfoil (seasoned as desired) and broiling the steak for 4 minutes. Remove the steak from the broil and tent it in the tinfoil to keep it warm.
- Combine the garlic, mustard, vinegar, and oil and whisk well to combine thoroughly. Toss the lettuce using half the dressing.
- Slice the steak and place it and the remaining ingredients on top of the tossed salad. Top with dressing prior to serving.

Orange Beef Stew

Makes enough for: 4
Time required for proper preparation: 15 minutes
Suggested cooking time: 8 hours
Total required: 8 hours and 15 minutes

What to Use
- Salt (as needed)
- Pepper (as needed)
- Rutabagas (3 spiralized)
- Sage (1 T chopped fine)
- Thyme (1 T chopped fine)
- Rosemary (1 T chopped fine)
- Bay leaves (2)
- Cinnamon (2 tsp. ground)
- Water (4 c)
- Balsamic vinegar (.25 c)
- Orange juice (.5 c)
- Orange zest (1 orange)
- Garlic (2 cloves minced)
- Celery (1 stalked diced)
- Carrot (1 diced)
- Onion (1 diced)
- Coconut oil (3 T)
- Beef stew meat (900 g cubed)

What to Do
- Add everything except for the sage, thyme, rutabagas, and rosemary to the slow cooker. Adjust the slow cooker temperature to low and leave it covered for 8 hours.
- About 10 minutes prior to serving remove the bay leaves and add in the remaining ingredients.

Beef and Shirataki Noodles

Makes enough for: 2
Time required for proper preparation: 10 minutes
Suggested cooking time: 10 minutes
Total required: 20 minutes

What to Use
- Black pepper (as desired)
- Yellow onion (.5)
- Mozzarella cheese (2 oz. shredded)
- Shirataki noodles (.5 c)
- Ground beef (.75 lbs.)
- Coconut oil (2 T)
- Water (.5 c)

What to Do
- Turn the Instant Pot cooker to sauté before adding in the coconut oil. Once it is heated, add in the onion and allow it to cook for approximately 5 minutes until it is brown and soft. Add in the beef and brown it as well.
- Add in the water and the shirataki noodles before turning the Instant Pot cooker to steam and letting the shirataki noodles cook for approximately 5 minutes or until done.
- Once the timer goes off, and in the cheese and let it melt slightly prior to serving.

Shepherd's Pie

Makes enough for: 12
Time required for proper preparation: 15 minutes
Suggested cooking time: 30 minutes
Total required: 45 minutes

What to Use
- Water (1 c)
- Coconut oil (4 T)
- Cauliflower (1 head)
- Cream cheese (4 oz.)
- Mozzarella (1 c)
- Egg (1)
- Salt (as desired)
- Pepper (as desired)
- Garlic powder (1 T)
- Ground beef (2 lbs.)
- Peas (1 c)
- Carrots (1 c)
- Mushrooms (8 oz. sliced)
- Beef broth (1 c)

What to Do

- Pour the water into the Instant Pot and arrange the cauliflower on top with the leaves and stems removed. Close the lid and set approximately 5 minutes or until done using high pressure.
- Quick release and add the cauliflower to a blender. Add the cream cheese, Coconut oil, mozzarella, egg, pepper, and salt. Blend until smooth.
- Drain the water from the Instant Pot. Toss in the beef, carrots, peas, garlic powder, and broth with a bit more pepper and salt to your liking.
- Blend in the cauliflower mixture and cook ten minutes on high (manual function).
- Serve and enjoy!

Cabbage Roll 'Unstuffed' Soup

Makes enough for: 9
Time required for proper preparation: 10 minutes
Suggested cooking time: 30 minutes
Total required: 40 minutes

What to Use
- Garlic (2 cloves minced)
- Onion (1 diced)
- Ground beef (1.5 lb.)
- Bragg's Aminos (.25 c)
- Tomato sauce (8 oz.)
- Beef broth (3 c.)
- Worcestershire sauce 'keto' approved/another substitute (3 t.)
- Diced tomatoes (14 oz.)
- Chopped cabbage (1)
- Parsley (.5 t)
- Pepper (as desired)
- Salt (as desired)

What to Do

- Add everything to the pressure cooker and mix well.
- Program the unit on the soup function. Natural release the soup for about ten minutes, and quick release the rest of the steam. Stir and serve.

Greek Meatballs with Tomato Sauce

Makes enough for: 6
Time required for proper preparation: 35 minutes
Suggested cooking time: 15 minutes
Total required: 50 minutes

What to Use - *Meatballs*
- Egg (1 slightly beaten)
- Ground beef (1 lb.)
- Chopped parsley (.25 c.)
- Finely chopped onion (.5 c.)
- Arborio rice (.3 c.)
- Salt (as desired)
- Pepper (as desired)

What to Use - *Sauce*
- Water (1 c)
- Tomatoes (14 oz. diced)
- Smoked paprika (.5 t)
- Cinnamon (.5 t)
- Dried oregano (1 t)
- Cloves (.25 t ground)
- Salt (as desired)
- Pepper (as desired)

What to Do

- Mix all of the meatballs fixings, shaping into eight to ten balls. Arrange in a single layer in the pot.
- Mix the sauce components in a dish and pour over the prepared meatballs.
- Program the Instant Pot for 15 minutes under high-pressure and release the pressure with the natural release option.
- Remove the meatballs and blend the sauce until smooth with an immersion blender. Pour over the meatballs, garnish, and serve.

Bunless Burger

Makes enough for: 6
Time required for proper preparation: 35 minutes
Suggested cooking time: 15 minutes
Total required: 50 minutes

What to Use
- Grass-fed Ground Beef (1.5 lbs.)
- Pepper (as desired)
- Pepper Jack Cheese (4 thick slices)
- Bacon (8 slices)
- Large Red Onion, Sliced (1 total)
- Romaine Lettuce Leaves (8 total)
- Salt (as desired)

What to Do

- Warm ground beef to room temperature, and then shape beef into 4 patties. Use thumb to make an indent in the center of each patty, so they cook evenly.
- Take a broiler pan and place each patty, thumbprint side facing up. Season as desired and heat the oven's broiler to high. Once hot, place patties on the center rack and broil for 7 minutes.
- When done, the patties should be golden brown and cooked. Remove from oven and top with a slice of pepper jack cheese on each. Replace in oven and broil to thoroughly, taking care to watch for signs of doneness, so they don't burn.
- Add the bacon to the skillet before placing the skillet on top of a burner set to medium heat and let it cook as needed.

Stir Fry with Cabbage

Makes enough for: 4
Time required for proper preparation: 20 minutes
Suggested cooking time: 25 minutes
Total required: 45 minutes

What to Use
- Wasabi paste (.5 T)
- Keto mayonnaise (1 c)
- Sesame oil (1 T)
- Ginger (1 T grated)
- Chili flakes (1 tsp.)
- Scallions (3 sliced)
- Garlic (2 cloves)
- White wine vinegar (1 T)
- Black pepper (.25 tsp. ground)
- Onion powder (1 tsp.)
- Salt (1 tsp.)
- Beef (1.3 lbs. ground)
- Coconut oil (5 oz. grass fed)
- Cabbage (1.6 lbs. shredded)

What to Do
- Add 3 oz. coconut oil to a frying pan before placing the pan on a burner set to a high/medium heat.
- Add the cabbage to the frying pan and let it cook, taking care to prevent it from browning. Season using vinegar and spices before continuing to stir and fry an additional 2 minutes before removing the cabbage from heat.
- Add the remainder of the coconut oil to the frying pan before adding in the ginger, chili flakes, and garlic and sautéing for 3 minutes.
- Add in the meat and season using pepper, salt, and sesame oil and ensure everything is hot prior to serving.
- Combine the wasabi paste and the mayo and add the results to the stir fry prior to serving.

Ground Beef, Veggies, and Noodles

Makes enough for: 6
Time required for proper preparation: 10 minutes
Suggested cooking time: 10 minutes
Total required: 20 minutes

What to Use
- Oil (1 T)
- Ground beef (1 lb.)
- Bell peppers (1 c chopped)
- Garlic (2 cloves)
- Onion (.5 c chopped)
- Baby spinach (4 c)
- Shirataki noodles (2 packages)
- Parmesan cheese (.5 c grated)

What to Do
- Prepare the Instant Pot on the sauté function and add the oil when hot.
- Add the garlic, ground beef, onions, peppers, and spinach. Scrape the browning bits from the bottom and secure the lid.
- Use the high-pressure setting for three minutes and quick-release the pressure. Empty the sauce over the noodles and garnish with the cheese.

Chili

Makes enough for: 6
Time required for proper preparation: 25 minutes
Suggested cooking time: 3 hours
Total required: 3 hours and 25 minutes

What to Use

- Worcestershire sauce (1 tsp.)
- Cayenne pepper (.5 tsp.)
- Oregano (1 tsp.)
- Paprika (2 tsp.)
- Garlic (2 tsp. minced)
- Fish sauce (2 tsp.)
- Cumin (1.5 tsp.)
- Chili powder (2 T + 1 tsp.)
- Coconut oil (2 T)
- Soy sauce (2 T)
- Tomato paste (.3 c)
- Beef broth (1 c)
- Green pepper (1 chopped)
- Onion (1 chopped)
- Ground beef (2 lbs.)

What to Do

- In a small bowl, combine the Worcestershire sauce, cayenne pepper, oregano, paprika, cumin, fish sauce, 2 T chili powder, and soy sauce and mix well to form a sauce.
- Add the garlic, green pepper and onion to a skillet before placing it on the stove over a burner turned to medium heat and letting them sauté until you can begin to see through the onions.
- Add everything to a slow cooker and combine thoroughly.
- Cover the slow cooker and let it cook on high heat for 2.5 hours and then uncovered for an additional 30 minutes.

Quarter Pound Burger

Makes enough for: 2
Time required for proper preparation: 10 minutes
Suggested cooking time: 8 minutes
Total required: 18 minutes

What to Use

- Basil (half a tsp.)
- Cayenne (fourth a tsp.)
- Crushed red pepper (half a tsp.)
- Salt (half a tsp.)
- Lettuce (2 large leaves)
- Coconut oil (2 T)
- Egg (1 large)
- Sriracha (1 T)
- Onion (fourth of whole onion)
- Plum tomato (half of a whole tomato)
- Mayo (1 T)
- Pickled jalapenos (1 T, sliced)
- Bacon (1 strip)
- Ground beef (.5 lbs.)
- Bacon (1 strip)

What to Do

- Knead mean for about three minutes.
- Chop bacon, jalapeno, tomato, and onion into fine pieces. (shown below)
- Knead in mayo, sriracha, egg, and chopped ingredients, and spices into the meat.
- Separate meat into four even pieces and flatten them (not thinly, just press on the tops to create a flat surface). Place a T of Coconut oil on top of two of the meat pieces. Take the pieces that do not have Coconut oil on them and set them on top of the coconut oiled ones (basically creating a Coconut oil and meat sandwich). Seal the sides together, concealing the coconut oil within.
- Throw the patties on the grill (or in a pan) for about 5 minutes on each side. Caramelize some onions if you want to!
- Prepare large leaves of lettuce by spreading some mayo onto them. Once patties are finished, place them on one half of the lettuce, add your desired burger toppings, and fold the other half over the lettuce leaf over the patty.
- Burger time!

Brussel Sprouts and Hamburger

Makes enough for: 3
Time required for proper preparation: 30 minutes
Suggested cooking time: 15 minutes
Total required: 45 minutes

What to Use
- Black pepper (as desired)
- Sea salt (as desired)
- Italian seasoning (1 T)
- Shredded cheese (5.3 oz.)
- Coconut oil (2 oz.)
- Sour cream (4 T)
- Brussel sprouts (1 lb. halved)
- Bacon (oz. diced)
- Ground beef (1 lb.)

What to Do
- Ensure your oven is heated to 425F.
- Add the Brussel sprouts and bacon to a frying pan and place the pan on the stove over a burner turned to high/medium. Season before adding in the sour cream and add the results to the baking dish.
- Add in the ground beef, herbs, and cheese.
- Add the baking sheet to oven and let it cook for 15 minutes.

Beef Casserole

Makes enough for: 4
Time required for proper preparation: 20 minutes
Suggested cooking time: 25 minutes
Total required: 45 minutes

What to Use
- Black pepper (as desired)
- Sea salt (as desired)
- Guacamole (1 c)
- Coconut oil (2 oz.)
- Scallion (1 chopped fine)
- Crème Fraiche (1 c)
- Cheese (7 oz. shredded)
- Jalapenos (2 oz.)
- Tomatoes (7 oz. crushed)
- Ground beef (1.5 lbs.)
- Cayenne pepper (1 pinch)
- Onion powder (1 tsp.)
- Garlic powder (1 tsp.)
- Cumin (1 tsp. ground)
- Paprika powder (2 tsp.)
- Chili powder (2 tsp.)

What to Do
- Ensure your oven is heated to 400F.
- Add the beef and tomatoes to a pan before placing it on the stove over a burner turned to a high/medium heat and then top with all the seasonings and mix well.
- Add the results to the baking dish before topping with the cheese and jalapenos. Place the dish on the top rack of the oven and let it bake approximately 20 minutes.
- Top with sour cream and chives and serve with guacamole.

Low-Carb Meatballs

Makes enough for: 2
Time required for proper preparation: 15 minutes
Suggested cooking time: 8 minutes
Total required: 23 minutes

What to Use
- Black pepper (as desired)
- Mozzarella cheese (.25 c)
- Garlic (1 T minced)
- Parmesan cheese (.25 c grated)
- Ground beef (.5 lbs.)
- Coconut oil (4 T)

What to Do
- Combine everything together in a large bowl before forming the results into 4 meatballs (2 per serving).
- Turn the Instant Pot cooker to sauté before adding in the oil and allowing it to warm up fully.
- Cook each meatball for approximately 2 minutes per side.

Instant Pot Steak

Makes enough for: 2
Time required for proper preparation: 15 minutes
Suggested cooking time: 35 minutes
Total required: 50 minutes

What to Use
- Worcestershire sauce (1.5 tsp)
- Flank steak (1 lb.)
- ACV (2 T)
- Coconut oil (.25 c)
- Onion soup mix (1 T)

What to Do
- Set to sauté.
- Brown the steak on both sides.
- Add onion soup mix, coconut oil, Worcestershire, and vinegar.
- Lock and seal lid.
- Set to meat/stew for 35 minutes. Carefully release pressure.

Maple Brisket

Makes enough for: 2
Time required for proper preparation: 15 minutes
Suggested cooking time: 40 minutes
Total required: 55 minutes

What to Use
- Beef brisket (1 lb.)
- Maple sugar (1 T)
- Pepper (as desired)
- Onion powder (.5 tsp.)
- Paprika (.25 tsp.)
- Mustard powder (.5 tsp.)
- Beef broth (1 c)
- Liquid smoke (1.5 tsp.)
- Thyme sprigs (2)

What to Do
- Mix dry spices together and coat brisket.
- Set pot to sauté. Grease with oil and brown brisket. Lay brisket fat side up, and add thyme, broth, and liquid smoke.
- Cook on high for 40 minutes. Once finished, let pressure release naturally. Remove and cover with foil.
- Optional: Turn to sauté and reduce leftover liquid.
- Slice brisket and drizzle with liquid.

Rosemary Veal

Makes enough for: 2
Time required for proper preparation: 15 minutes
Suggested cooking time: 5 hours
Total required: 5 hours and 15 minutes

What to Use
- Leg of lamb (1)
- Rosemary (2 sticks fresh)
- Pumpkin (1 medium quartered)
- Potatoes (2 c chopped)
- Carrots (2 sliced)
- Celery (1 stock sliced)
- Shallot (1 sliced)
- Vegetable broth (.75 c)
- Garlic (2 cloves sliced)
- Rosemary (.25 tsp dried)
- Coconut oil (.5 tsp)
- Whole wheat flour (2 tsp)
- Dijon mustard (1 tsp)
- Salt (as desired)
- Pepper (as desired)

What to Do
- You can cook this recipe either inside of your oven or in a slow cooker. If you decide to cook in an oven, you should increase the stock you use by up to 1 or 1.5 c and then also reduce the cooking time between either 1.5 hours or 2 hours than what you would in a slow cooker. For oven cooking, cook at 285F.
- To get started with your seasoned oil, cook on low heat in a frying pan so that the garlic and the shallot start to sizzle but do not turn brown. Next, remove the garlic and shallot and throw them away. Keep the remaining oil in the pan.
- Add in the vegetables in order to sauté them. Cook the vegetables until they start to appear brown over medium heat. You will then remove the vegetables and then place them inside the slow cooker if you choose to use one for this recipe.
- Next, remove any fat pieces from the lamb and then cut small slits in the meat. Use salt and pepper in order to season the meat, and then insert the sprigs of rosemary.
- Brown the lamb in your seasoned oil. You will then place the veal on top of the prepared vegetables that are resting inside the slow cooker. You should save a stick of rosemary and then break it into two pieces to place on both sides of the lamb.

- Mix together the flour and the mustard together, and then add it into the stock with the vegetables and veal. You will want to stir the mixture together until it becomes thick.
- Depending on the size of your veal, you should set your slow cooker between 4 or 5 hours to cook.

Beef Tenderloin with Couscous

Makes enough for: 2
Time required for proper preparation: 30 minutes
Suggested cooking time: 2 hours and 30 minutes
Total required: 3 hours

What to Use - *Beef*
- Beef tenderloin (2 fillets)
- Coconut oil (2 T)
- Pepper (as desired)
- Salt (as desired)

What to Use - *Couscous*
- Whole wheat couscous (1 c)
- Cherry tomatoes (2 halved)
- Shallot (1)
- Coconut oil (1 T)
- Lemon juice (2 tsp.)
- Cumin (1 tsp. ground)
- Chickpeas (14 oz.)
- Parsley (2 T freshly chopped)
- Salt (as desired)
- Pepper (as desired)

What to Do
- Drain and rinse the chickpeas.
- Set the Sous Vide Supreme to 130F (med-rare).
- Sprinkle the steaks with the pepper and salt. Seal each one in its own bag.
- Add them to the bath – not touching.
- Cover for 2 to 2.5 hours. When done, transfer them to a pan coated in the oil. Let them rest a few minutes before slicing.
- Make the couscous and combine with the chickpeas, tomatoes, coconut oil, lemon juice, and parsley. Sprinkle with the pepper and salt.
- Spoon the couscous onto a plate or bowl and top with the beef.
- Garnish with parsley and lemon slices.

Beef Tenderloin with Pesto and Asparagus

Makes enough for: 4
Time required for proper preparation: 20 minutes
Suggested cooking time: 20 minutes
Total required: 40 minutes

What to Use
- Beef tenderloin (4, 6 oz. pieces)
- Kosher salt – divided (1 T)
- Black pepper (as desired)
- Coconut oil (.25 c.)
- Garlic cloves (5 large)
- Parmesan cheese (2 T grated)
- Lemon (1 zest and juice)
- Asparagus spears (16-20)
- Basil leaves (1 c. fresh)

What to Do
- Set the temperature in the water bath to 135F.
- Sprinkle the meat with pepper and salt and place into two pouches. Vacuum seal. Set the timer for two hours.
- In boiling water on the stovetop, blanch the basil for 30 seconds. Transfer it to an ice bath. Drain and chop. Do the same for the garlic (30 seconds, and dip).
- Combine the basil, garlic, parmesan cheese, and one tsp of salt, along with the oil in a blender until smooth.
- Add the juice and adjust to your liking.
- Add the asparagus to a cooking bag in a single layer. Season with salt if desired and add a bit of the pesto. Vacuum seal and cook beside the meat for 15 minutes.
- Remove the packs and sear the meat for 30-45 seconds per side on a well-greased grill.
- Enjoy with the asparagus and more pesto.

Chapter 7: Vegan Recipes

Zoodles

Several of the recipes in this chapter center around zoodles. Zoodles are simply zucchini in the shape of noodles. They will allow you to enjoy all of your favorite pasta recipes without the carbs. These "noodles" are low in calories and carbs, yet they will taste just as delicious as any other noodle you could try. Plus, they can be made very quickly, ready to serve in minutes, or as a part of meal prep. You will want to ensure that the sauces you choose to use have high amounts of fat and protein to make up most of the energy from this meal, as zucchini alone is not high in either.

Makes enough for: 2
Time required for proper preparation: 5 minutes
Suggested cooking time: 0 minutes
Total required: 5 minutes

What to Use

*   Zucchini (4 organic)

What to Do - Zoodle Creation

*   If you have access to a spiralizer, use it to create noodles of zucchini. If you do not own a spiralizer, this recipe is still very simple. Just slice the zucchini into long thin strips. You may also wish to use a cheese and vegetable grater to get the desired noodle effect.
*   Serve the zoodles as they are, or let them boil for two minutes in a pan of water to warm them up and soften them a bit. Alternately, you may wish to sauté them in a bit of coconut oil or Coconut oil for a minute or two to give them a little crispness.
*   Serve the zoodles in place of the traditional noodles in your favorite pasta dishes.

Biryani

Makes enough for: 6
Time required for proper preparation: 15 minutes
Suggested cooking time: 15 minutes
Total required: 30 minutes

What to Use
- Black pepper (as desired)
- Sea salt (as desired)
- Garam masala (.5 tsp)
- Coconut oil (1 tsp)
- Shelled peas (1 c)
- Water (2.5 c)
- Coriander (.5 tsp ground)
- Chili powder (1 tsp)
- Turmeric (1.5 tsp)
- Carrots (2 quartered)
- Potatoes (2 quartered)
- Bay leaves (2 torn)
- Cumin seeds (.5 tsp)
- Onion (1 sliced thin)
- Vegetable oil (3 T)
- White rice long grain (2 c)

What to Do
- Add the rice to a large pot and cover it with three to four inches of water before allowing it to soak for about 20 minutes. Drain and set aside.
- Add the oil to your pressure cooker and set it over medium heat. Add in the onion, bay leaves, and cumin seeds and let everything cook for about 5 minutes until the onion is nearly see through.
- Mix in the carrots and potatoes and let them cook for an additional 5 minutes and the potatoes have begun to brown. Add in the coriander, turmeric and chili powder and let everything cook for 1 additional minute.
- Add the rice to the pressure cooker and ensure it is well covered in the boil before adding in the peas and water. Mix in the garam masala, oil, and salt before sealing the cooker and turning it to high pressure. Let everything cook for 5 minutes before removing from heat.
- Allow the pressure to naturally release and fluff the rice with a fork prior to serving.

Greek Mixed Roasted Vegetables

Makes enough for: 4
Time required for proper preparation: 15 minutes
Suggested cooking time: 45 minutes
Total required: 60 minutes

What to Use - Vegetables
- 1 eggplant (peeled and diced .75-inch
- Black pepper(as desired)
- Kosher sea salt (as desired)
- Extra virgin olive oil (2 T)
- Garlic (2 cloves minced)
- Onion (1 peeled, diced 1-inch)
- Bell pepper (2 red, yellow, diced, 1-inch)

What to Use - Dressing
- Coconut oil (.25 c)
- Lemon juice (.3 c squeezed fresh)
- Black pepper (as desired)
- Kosher sea salt (as desired)
- Basil (15 leaves)
- Scallions (4 minced)

What to Do
- Ensure your oven is heated to 425F.
- One a sheet pan, combine the garlic, onion, yellow bell pepper, red bell pepper, and eggplant before seasoning using the pepper, salt, and coconut oil.
- Add the pan to the oven and let it cook for 40 minutes, using a spatula to flip everything after 20 minutes.
- As the vegetables are cooking, combine the pepper, salt, coconut oil, and lemon juice together in a small bowl, add the results to the vegetables as soon as they are ready.
- Let the pan cool completely before adding in the basil, feta, and scallions. Season prior to serving.

Autumn Roasted Green Beans

Makes enough for: 4
Time required for proper preparation: 15 minutes
Suggested cooking time: 30 minutes
Total required: 45 minutes

What to Use
- Walnuts (.5 c toasted)
- Cranberries (.5 c dried)
- Black pepper (as desired)
- Kosher sea salt (as desired)
- Lemon juice (2 tsp.)
- Lemon zest (1 tsp.)
- Sugar (.25 tsp.)
- Coconut oil (2 T)
- Garlic (4 cloves, quartered and peeled)
- Green beans (2 lbs. stems trimmed)

What to Do
- Preheat your oven to 350F and crack and smash the walnuts into chunks.
- Spread the walnuts onto a baking sheet and toast them for 10 minutes.
- Increase the temperature on the oven to 450F.
- Cover a baking sheet with a rim using aluminum foil.
- In a mixing bowl, combine the sugar, pepper, salt and coconut oil before coating the garlic and green beans thoroughly.
- Place the beans onto a baking sheet and spread them out to ensure they cook well. Place the sheet into the oven and let the beans bake for 15 minutes before stirring with a spatula and roasting another 10 minutes.
- Mix in the lemon juice, pepper and salt prior to serving.

Roasted Summer Squash

Makes enough for: 4
Time required for proper preparation: 5 minutes
Suggested cooking time: 30 minutes
Total required: 35 minutes

What to Use
- Zucchini (3)
- Yellow squash (3)
- Kosher salt (1.5 T)
- Black pepper (.5 T)
- Coconut oil (2 T)

What to Do
- Ensure your oven is heated to 400F
- Peel vegetables and cut into .25 inch thick slices.
- Assemble vegetables on a baking sheet or pan and drizzle coconut oil on top. Sprinkle with seasoning as desired
- Bake at 400F for 30 minutes.

Savory Baked Acorn Squash

Makes enough for: 4
Time required for proper preparation: 5 minutes
Suggested cooking time: 30 minutes
Total required: 35 minutes

What to Use
- Acorn squash (1)
- Kosher salt (as desired)
- Black pepper (as desired)
- Coconut oil (2 tsp.)
- Smoked paprika (as desired)

What to Do
- Ensure your oven is heated to 425F.
- Cut acorn squash in half lengthwise, then cut halves into quarters lengthwise. Scoop out seeds and discard.
- Place the squash on baking sheet and drizzle coconut oil over the top of each quarter. Scatter with the smoked paprika, salt, and pepper and bake in the oven for 30 minutes.

Roasted Brussels Sprouts

Makes enough for: 4
Time required for proper preparation: 5 minutes
Suggested cooking time: 15 minutes
Total required: 20 minutes

What to Use
- Sea salt (.25 tsp.)
- Black pepper (.25 tsp.)
- Brussel sprouts (.75lbs. sliced in half length-wise)
- Coconut oil (1.5 T.)

What to Do
- Ensure your oven is heated to 400F. Cut Brussels sprouts in half and place in a medium-sized bowl. Drizzle the coconut oil over the Brussels sprouts and then toss with the sea salt and black pepper until evenly coated.
- Pour Brussels sprouts onto a baking sheet and make sure they are evenly spaced so that they will roast easily.
- Place the sheet in the oven and let it cook for approximately 10 minutes before stirring well and returning it to the oven for 10 minutes more. Season as desired. They will keep in the fridge for 3-4 days or in the freezer for 2-3 months.

Roasted Rosemary Potatoes

Makes enough for: 6
Time required for proper preparation: 10 minutes
Suggested cooking time: 25 minutes
Total required: 35 minutes

What to Use
- Garlic (1 head)
- Rosemary (3 sprigs)
- Thyme (3 sprigs)
- Baby potatoes (20 oz.)
- Parsley (2 T chopped)
- Sea salt (as desired)
- Black pepper (as desired)
- Coconut oil (2 T)

What to Do
- Ensure your oven is heated to 450F.
- Separate garlic cloves and remove the papery skin, holding them together, but do not peel.
- Add the rosemary, thyme, baby potatoes, parsley, garlic, and coconut oil together in a large bowl, coating well.
- Add the results to a jelly roll pan that has been lined with tinfoil before topping with pepper and salt. Place the pan in the oven and let the potatoes bake for approximately 25 minutes, stirring at the 12-minute mark.
- Season with additional pepper and salt prior to serving.

Sweet Potato Wedges

Makes enough for: 6
Time required for proper preparation: 10 minutes
Suggested cooking time: 30 minutes
Total required: 40 minutes

What to Use
- Salt (1 tsp.)
- Cracked black pepper (1 tsp.)
- Garlic powder (.5 tsp.)
- Sweet potatoes (4 medium, peeled, each cut into 6 wedges
- Rosemary (1 T chopped, fresh)
- Coconut oil (2 T)

What to Do
- Preheat oven to 450F.
- In a mixing bowl, combine the coconut oil, rosemary, sweet potatoes, garlic powder, black pepper, and salt together and ensure the potatoes are coated well.
- Add the results in a single layer to a large roasting pan before placing the pan in the oven and letting the potatoes bake for 20 minutes. Turn the dish at this point before baking another 10 minutes.

Best Lentil Curry

Makes enough for: 4
Time required for proper preparation: 10 min
Suggested cooking time: 30 minutes
Total required: 40 minutes

What to Use
- Vegetable broth (4 c low sodium)
- Red lentil (1 c)
- Potato (10 oz. peeled and made into pieces that are 1 inch each)
- Carrot (8 oz. chopped)
- Curry powder (1 T)
- Scallions (8 separated, sliced)
- Garlic (2 cloves chopped)
- Ginger (2 T chopped)
- Coconut oil (3 T)

What to Do
- Add the oil to a saucepan before placing it on the stove on top of a burner set to a high/medium heat.
- Add in the scallion whites, garlic and ginger and let them soften for 2 minutes.
- Mix in the curry powder as well as pepper and salt, as desired, broth, lentils, potato, and carrots before letting everything boil. Turn down the heat and let everything simmer for 15 minutes, stirring regularly.
- Top with scallion greens prior to serving.

Chana Masala

Makes enough for: 4
Time required for proper preparation: 5 minutes
Suggested cooking time: 25 minutes
Total required: 30 minutes

What to Use
- Curry powder (1 tsp.)
- Chickpeas (32 oz. rinsed, drained)
- Garlic (2 cloves minced)
- Onion (1 large, chopped)
- Extra virgin olive oil (1 T)
- Cilantro (.25 c)
- Kosher sea salt (as desired)
- Lemon juice (1 T)
- Tomatoes (2 chopped)
- Ginger (2 tsp. grated)
- Turmeric (.5 tsp.)

What to Do
- Add the oil to a skillet before placing it on a burner set to a medium/high heat. Add in the onion and let it sauté until it has become translucent and soft. Mix in the garlic and let it cook for 3 minutes.
- Add in the curry powder, chickpeas, coconut oil, lemon juice, tomatoes, ginger and turmeric, along with .25 c of water. Let the mixture simmer before cooking it for 10 minutes, stirring on occasion. The end result should have a stew-like consistency but not be runny.
- Season using salt and top with cilantro prior to serving.

Zucchini Noodle Pasta with Avocado Pesto

Makes enough for: 8
Time required for proper preparation: 30 minutes
Suggested cooking time: 15 minutes
Total required: 45 hour

What to Use
- Zucchinis (6 spiralized)
- Cold pressed oil of choice (1 T)

What to Use - Pesto
- Pine nuts (.25 c)
- Avocados (2 cubed)
- Parsley (.25 c leaves)
- Basil (1 c leaves)
- Garlic (3 cloves)
- Lemon juice (1 lemon)
- Cold pressed oil of choice (3 T)
- Salt (as desired)
- Pepper (as desired)

What to Do
- Spiralize your zucchini and set aside on paper towels.
- In a food processor, add in all ingredients for the avocado pesto except the oil. Pulse on low until desired consistency is reached.
- Slowly add in coconut oil until creamy and emulsified.
- Heat 1 T and your zucchini noodles cook for 4 min.
- Take your zucchini noodles and coat with avocado pesto.

Thai Soup

Makes enough for: 9
Time required for proper preparation: 30 minutes
Suggested cooking time: 15 minutes
Total required: 45 hour

What to Use
- Spiralized Zucchinis (2 medium)
- Minced Garlic Cloves (2 total)
- Thin Sliced Red Pepper (1 total)
- Diced Jalapeno (1 total)
- Lime (1 cut into 8 wedges)
- Thin Sliced Onion (0.5 total)
- Full-Fat Coconut Milk (15oz)
- Vegetable Broth (6 c)
- Fresh Chopped Cilantro (0.5 c)
- Green Curry Paste (1.5 T)
- Coconut Oil (1 T)

What to Do
- Add the coconut oil to a saucepan before adding in the onions and letting them sauté. Takes about 5 minutes.
- Add jalapeno, curry paste, and minced garlic. Sauté for 1 minute or until just fragrant. Stir in bone broth and coconut milk, mix until thoroughly combined. Heat until soup comes to a boil and then reduce to medium heat. Add red pepper slices, then mix.
- Simmer soup approximately 5 minutes or until done, until chicken is cooked through. Add fresh cilantro.
- Divide zucchini into 8 bowls and ladle soup over them. The heat of the soup will cook the zucchini noodles. If not serving all at once, store soup and zoodles separately and combine when prepared to eat, so zoodles don't become soggy.

Vegan Lasagna

Makes enough for: 8
Time required for proper preparation: 10 minutes
Suggested cooking time: 4 hours
Total required: 4 hours and 10 minutes

What to Use
- Lasagna Zoodles (6)
- Vegan cheese (2.5 c)
- Red pepper flakes (.25 tsp.)
- Basil (.5 tsp. dried)
- Oregano (1 tsp. dried)
- Salt (1 tsp.)
- Tomato sauce (15 oz.)
- Tomato (28 oz. crushed)
- Garlic (1 clove minced)
- Onion (1 chopped)
- Ground soy (1 lb.)

What to Do
- Place a skillet on the stove on top of a burner set to a high/medium heat before adding in the garlic, onion, and soy and letting the soy brown.
- Add in the red pepper flakes, basil, oregano, salt, tomato sauce, and crushed tomatoes and let the results simmer for 5 minutes.
- Add .3 of the total sauce from the skillet and add it to the slow cooker. Place 3 Zoodles on top of the sauce, followed by the cheese mixture. Create three layers in total.
- Cover the slow cooker and let it cook on a low heat for 6 hours.

Caprese Zoodles

Makes enough for: 4
Time required for proper preparation: 10 minutes
Suggested cooking time: 15 minutes
Total required: 25 minutes

What to Use
- Zucchini (4 large)
- 2 T coconut oil
- Kosher salt (as desired)
- Black pepper (as desired)
- Cherry tomatoes, (2 c halved)
- Mozzarella balls (1 c quartered)
- Basil leaves (.25 c torn)
- Balsamic vinegar (2 T)

What to Do
- Place the zoodles in a serving bowl before adding in the coconut oil and tossing well. Season as desired and allow the zoodles to marinate for at least 15 minutes.
- Mix in the basil, mozzarella, and tomatoes and toss well.
- Top with balsamic prior to serving.

Burrito Zoodles

Makes enough for: 4
Time required for proper preparation: 25 minutes
Suggested cooking time: 15 minutes
Total required: 40 minutes

What to Use
- Coconut oil (2 T)
- Onion (1 medium, chopped)
- Garlic (2 cloves minced)
- Chili powder (1 tsp.)
- Cumin (.5 tsp. ground)
- Kosher salt (as desired)
- Black pepper(as desired)
- Black beans (15 oz. drained and rinsed)
- Cherry tomatoes (1 c halved)
- Red enchilada sauce (1 c)
- Cheddar (1 c shredded)
- Monterey Jack (1 c shredded)
- Zoodles (14 oz.)

What to Do
- Add the oil to the skillet before placing it on the stove over a burner turned to medium heat.
- Add in the carrot and onion and allow both to cook approximately 5 minutes before adding in the garlic and allowing it to cook for approximately 60 seconds.
- Mix in the cumin, chili powder, salt, and pepper before adding in the cheese, enchilada sauce, cherry tomatoes, and black beans.
- Allow everything to simmer for approximately 10 minutes before adding in the zoodles and tossing to coat. Let the zoodles cook for approximately 3 minutes, stirring regularly.

Red Pepper Zoodles

Makes enough for: 4
Time required for proper preparation: 10 minutes
Suggested cooking time: 25 minutes
Total required: 35 minutes

What to Use
- Red bell peppers (1)
- Almond milk (1 c)
- Coconut oil (1 T)
- Salt (1 tsp.)
- Garlic (1 clove)
- Almond Coconut oil (.25 c)

What to Do
- Prepare a baking sheet by lining it with foil.
- Add the bell peppers to the baking sheet before placing them on the top level of your broiler and letting them cook until blackened.
- Once they have cooled, you can remove the skins, stems, seeds, and ribs.
- Add the results, along with the remaining sauce ingredients and blend thoroughly. Season as desired.
- Serve with zoodles as well as a variety of potential toppings, including things like truffle oil, goat cheese, parmesan cheese or parsley.

Zoodles Marinara

Makes enough for: 4
Time required for proper preparation: 15 minutes
Suggested cooking time: 15 minutes
Total required: 30 minutes

What to Use
- Extra virgin coconut oil (2 T)
- White onions (.5 c diced)
- Garlic cloves (6 minced)
- Tomatoes (14 oz. diced)
- Tomato paste (2 T)
- Basil leaves (.5 c roughly-chopped loosely packed)
- Coarse salt (1.5 tsp)
- Black pepper (.25 tsp)
- Cayenne (1 pinch)
- Zucchinis (2 large spiralized)
- Parmesan cheese (as desired)

What to Do
- Add the oil to the skillet before placing it on the stove over a burner turned to a medium heat.
- Add in the onion and allow it to cook approximately 5 minutes before adding in the garlic and allowing it to cook for approximately 60 seconds.
- Mix in the crushed red pepper flakes, pepper, salt, basil tomato paste, and tomatoes and combine thoroughly.
- Allow the sauce to simmer before reducing the heat to medium/low. Let the sauce simmer an additional 15 minutes or until the oil takes on a deep orange color, which indicates the sauce is thickened and reduced. Season as desired.
- Add in the zoodles and let them soften for approximately 2 minutes.
- Top with parmesan cheese prior to serving.

Zoodle Japchae

Makes enough for: 2
Time required for proper preparation: 15 minutes
Suggested cooking time: 8 minutes
Total required: 23 minutes

What to Use
- Spinach (2.5 c packed)
- Coconut oil (1 T)
- Carrot (1 halved)
- White onion (.5 sliced thin)
- Shitake mushrooms (3.5 oz. sliced)
- Zucchini (1 sliced)
- Sesame oil (1 T)
- Honey (2 tsp.)
- Soy sauce (2 T)

What to Do
- Fill a small pot with water before placing it on the stove over a burner turned to high heat.
- While waiting for the pot to boil, combine the soy sauce, honey, sesame oil in a small bowl, whisk well and set to one side.
- After the water, boils add in the spinach and let it cook until it begins to wilt. Remove it from the water with the help of a slotted spoon and squeeze out any excess water.
- Add the oil to the skillet before placing it on the stove over a burner turned to medium heat.
- Add in the onion, carrot and shitake mushrooms before allowing them to cook approximately 5 minutes.
- Add in the zoodles and toss approximately 2 minutes. Add the results to a colander and toss to remove excess moisture.
- Return the zoodles to the skillet, add in the spinach and top with the sauce. Toss for approximately 60 seconds.

Chapter 8: Snack Recipes

Olive and Tomato Balls

Makes enough for: 5
Time required for proper preparation: 10 minutes
Suggested cooking time: 35 minutes
Total required: 45 minutes

What to Use
- Parmesan cheese (5 T grated)
- Salt (.25 tsp.)
- Black pepper (as desired)
- Garlic (2 cloves crushed)
- Kalamata olives (4 pitted)
- Sun-dried tomatoes (4 pieces drained)
- Oregano (2 T chopped)
- Thyme (2 T chopped)
- Basil (2 T chopped)
- Coconut oil (.25 c)
- Cream cheese (.5 c)

What to Do
- Chop the coconut oil and add it to a small mixing bowl with the cream cheese and leave them both to soften for about 30 minutes. Mash together and mix well to combine.
- Add in the Kalamata olives and sun-dried tomatoes and mix well before adding in the herbs and seasonings. Combine thoroughly before placing the mixing bowl in the refrigerator to allow the results to solidify.
- Once it has solidified, form the mixture into a total of 5 balls using an ice cream scoop. Roll each of the finished balls into the parmesan cheese before plating.
- Extras can be stored in the refrigerator in an air-tight container for up to 7 days.

Brown Rice Pilaf

Makes enough for: 4
Time required for proper preparation: 20 minutes
Suggested cooking time: 30 minutes
Total required: 50 minutes

What to Use
- Black pepper (as desired)
- Sea salt (as desired)
- Cashews (.25 c chopped)
- Parsley (.25 c chopped)
- Eggs (2 beaten)
- Chickpeas (1 c)
- Mushrooms (2 c sliced)
- Carrots (2 sliced)
- Garlic (1 clove minced)
- Onion (1.5 c chopped)
- Coconut oil (3 T)
- Brown rice (.75 c)
- Water (1.5 c)

What to Do
- Add 1.5 c water to a pot before placing the pot on the stove on top of a burner turned to high heat. Once it comes to a boil, add in the rice; once it comes back to a boil, turn the heat to lower, cover the pot and allow the rice to simmer for about 45 minutes or until the rice reaches your desired level of tenderness.
- Some 15 minutes before the rice has finished simmering, add the coconut oil to a skillet before adding the pan to the stove on top of a burner turned to medium heat. Add in the onions and allow them to sauté, stirring frequently until they are soft. Mix in the carrots and garlic and stir regularly for approximately 5 minutes or until done.
- Add the mushrooms to the skillet and allow them to brown for about 10 minutes before adding in the chickpeas and cooking for an additional 60 seconds.
- After the rice has finished cooking, add the eggs into the skillet and let the eggs cook, stirring constantly. Remove the skillet from the burner before adding in the nuts, parsley, and pepper prior to serving.

Easy Sheet Pan Roasted Vegetables

Makes enough for: 8
Time required for proper preparation: 20 minutes
Suggested cooking time: 25 minutes
Total required: 45 minutes

What to Use
- Pepper (.25 tsp.)
- Red onion (1 chopped)
- Balsamic vinegar (1 T)
- Coarse salt (1 tsp.)
- Red bell peppers (2 chopped)
- Italian seasoning (2 tsp.)
- Cubed Coconut oilnut squash (3 C)
- Extra virgin coconut oil (3 T)
- Broccoli florets (4 C)

What to Do
- Ensure your oven is preheated to 425F.
- Toss cubed squash in a T of oil and spread out onto a baking tray. Roast for 10 minutes.
- Toss pepper, salt, Italian seasoning, onion, bell peppers, and broccoli till coated well.
- Add roasted squash to the veggies. Toss well to incorporate. Spread veggie mixture over two baking trays.
- Roast 17 to 20 minutes, making sure to stir around 1-2 times throughout the cooking process. Vegetables should be tender and browned in areas.
- Drizzle with vinegar before eating.
- Can be refrigerated for up to 7 days.

Asian Mason Jar Salad

Makes enough for: 4
Time required for proper preparation: 15 minutes
Suggested cooking time: 0 minutes
Total required: 15 minutes

What to Use - *Salad*
- Snap peas (1.3 c halved)
- Cucumber (1.3 c sliced)
- Carrots (1.3 c grated)
- Unsalted cashews (1 c)
- Red pepper (1 julienned)
- Baby spinach (2 c sliced)
- Napa cabbage (2 c sliced)
- Rotisserie chicken (2 c shredded)
- Green onions (2 T sliced)

What to Use - *Dressing*
- Garlic clove (1 minced)
- Honey (1 T)
- Ginger (1 T minced)
- Coconut oil (1 T)
- Sesame seeds (1 tsp.)
- Sriracha sauce (1 tsp.)
- Toasted sesame oil (2.5 T)
- Cilantro (2 T)
- Rice vinegar (2 T)
- Low-sodium soy sauce (3 T)

What to Do
- Whisk sesame seeds, honey, cilantro, garlic, ginger, sriracha, coconut oil, toasted sesame oil, vinegar, and soy sauce together.
- Toss spinach and Napa cabbage together.
- Assemble jars by add three T of dressing, .3 C snap peas, .25 C chicken, .25 C cashews, and a sprinkle of green onion. Serve now or place in the fridge.

Parmesan Zucchini Tomato Gratin

Makes enough for: 6
Time required for proper preparation: 10 minutes
Suggested cooking time: 40 minutes
Total required: 50 minutes

What to Use
- Basil (2 tsp.)
- Garlic powder (1 tsp.)
- Salt (.5 tsp.)
- Garlic (2 T minced)
- Coconut oil (2 T)
- Onion (.5 c chopped)
- Parmesan cheese (.5 c shredded)
- Tomatoes (2)
- Zucchini (3)

What to Do
- Ensure your oven is preheated to 350F.
- Sauté onions until translucent and fragrant. Add garlic, sautéing 1 to 2 minutes longer. Pour mixture into the bottom of a casserole dish.
- With a knife, slice tomatoes and zucchinis.
- Layer zucchini and tomatoes, alternating layers.
- Drizzle veggies with coconut oil, sprinkle with seasonings and cover with Parmesan cheese.
- Bake 40 minutes until gratin turns a light brown.

Spicy Deviled Eggs

Makes enough for: 6
Time required for proper preparation: 30 minutes
Suggested cooking time: 0 minutes
Total required: 30 minutes

What to Use
- Smoked paprika (.25 tsp.)
- Cream cheese (2 oz. softened)
- Mayonnaise (4 T)
- Bacon (6 slices cooked, crumbled)
- Pickled jalapenos (16 sliced, divided)
- Egg (6)

What to Do
- In a large saucepan, add in the eggs before filling the pan with enough water that the eggs are submerged under 1 inch of water.
- Add the pan to the stove over a saucepan turned to high heat. After the water boils, remove the pan from the stove and let the contents cool for 12 minutes.
- Peel the eggs and cut them in half vertically.
- Add the yolks to a mixing bowl and mash well. Add in the jalapenos, cream cheese, mayonnaise, and bacon.
- Add the results to each of the egg halves, chill, serve and enjoy.

Granola

Makes enough for: 12
Time required for proper preparation: 20 minutes
Suggested cooking time: 2 hours
Total required: 2 hours and 20 minutes

What to Use
- Swerve (.5c)
- Salt (1 tsp.)
- Pumpkin seeds (1 c)
- Raw almonds (.5c)
- Raw walnuts (.5c)
- Vanilla extract (1 tsp.)
- Raw pecans (.5c)
- Raw hazelnuts (.5c)
- Raw sunflower seeds (1 c)
- Vanilla Stevia (1 tsp)
- Ground cinnamon (1 tsp)
- Unsweetened shredded coconut (1 c)
- Coconut oil (.3 c)

What to Do
- Set the cooker to sauté, then add the coconut oil and melt. When melted, add the vanilla extract and Stevia. Stir well before adding coconut, seeds, and nuts. Stir mixture well to coat all ingredients.
- In a bowl, whisk salt, cinnamon, and swerve, then sprinkle with seeds and nuts.
- Close and seal the lid. Set on slow cook on low for two hours and stir every 30 minutes.
- When done, quick-release the pressure. Spread onto a baking pan to cool and store in an airtight container.

Walnut Orange Chocolate Bombs

Makes enough for: 8
Time required for proper preparation: 3 hours and 30 minutes
Suggested cooking time: 0 minutes
Total required: 3 hours and 30 minutes

What to Use
- Extra virgin coconut oil (.25 c)
- Orange peel or orange extract (.5 T)
- Walnuts (1.75 c chopped)
- Cinnamon (1 tsp.)
- Stevia (10-15 drops)
- Cocoa dark chocolate (12 5g 85%)

What to Do
- Melt chocolate with your choice of method.
- Add cinnamon and coconut oil. Sweeten mixture with stevia.
- Pour in fresh orange peel and chopped walnuts.
- In a muffin tin or in candy c, spoon in mixture.
- Place into the fridge for 1-3 hours until mixture is solid.

Oatmeal Energy Bites

Makes enough for: 8
Time required for proper preparation: 5 minutes
Suggested cooking time: 10 minutes
Total required: 15 minutes

What to Use
- Flaxseed (.25 c ground)
- Chocolate chips (.5 c)
- Almond Coconut oil (.5 c)
- Rolled oats (1 c)
- Raw honey (.3 c)

What to Do
- Mix all recipe components together.
- Roll out tsp. sized balls onto a tray lined with parchment paper.
- Freeze balls for 1 hour.
- Freeze for up to 1 month.

Mini Pepper Nachos

Makes enough for: 8
Time required for proper preparation: 5 minutes
Suggested cooking time: 10 minutes
Total required: 15 minutes

What to Use
- Tomato (.5 c chopped)
- Chili powder (1 T)
- Cheddar cheese (shredded (1.5 c)
- Cumin (ground, 1 tsp.)
- Mini peppers (seeded, halved, 16 oz.)
- Garlic powder (1 tsp.)
- Ground beef (16 oz.)
- Paprika (1 tsp.)
- Red pepper flakes (.25 tsp.)
- Salt (kosher,.5 tsp.)
- Oregano (.5 tsp.)
- Pepper (.5 tsp.)

What to Do
- Mix seasonings together in a bowl.
- On medium heat, brown the meat, be sure all the clumps are broken up.
- Mix in the spices and continue to sauté until the seasoning has gone through all of the meat.
- Heat the oven to 400F.
- Place the peppers in a single line. They can touch.
- Coat with the beef mix.
- Sprinkle with cheese.
- Bake for around 10 minutes or until cheese has melted.
- Pull out of the oven and top with the toppings.

Cheesy Beef Balls

Makes enough for: 6
Time required for proper preparation: 50 minutes
Suggested cooking time: 20 minutes
Total required: 70 minutes

What to Use
- Cheddar (cubed, 12, optional)
- Ground beef (1.5 c)
- Cheddar cheese (shredded, 0.75 c)

What to Do
- Combine the beef and the cheese.
- Roll into twelve balls of equal size.
- If you are placing the cubed cheese in the middle, make sure that you do this before you roll them into balls.
- Deep fry them at 375F

Flaxseed Crackers and Keto Spinach and Artichoke Dip

Makes enough for: 6
Time required for proper preparation: 10 minutes
Suggested cooking time: 60 minutes
Total required: 70 minutes

What to Use
- Flax seeds (1 c)
- Red pepper flakes (.5 tsp., optional)
- Water (1 c)
- Onion powder (.5 tsp., optional)
- Rosemary (1 tsp., optional)
- Garlic powder (.5 tsp., optional)

What to Do
- Dump flax seeds into a bowl. Put in the fridge for up to eighteen hours.
- Take the flax seeds and place them on a sheet of parchment paper. Roll as thin as you can get them.
- Your oven needs to be set to 275F, and the seeds cooked for an hour on the paper they are sitting on.

Cream Cheese and Salmon Mug Muffin

Makes enough for: 1
Time required for proper preparation: 1.5 minutes
Suggested cooking time: 1.5 minutes
Total required: 3 minutes

What to Use
- Salt (as desired)
- Water (2 T)
- Cream (2 T)
- Egg (1 large)
- Baking soda (.25 tsp)
- Flax meal (.25 c)
- Almond flour (.25 c)
- Chives or scallions (2 T chopped)
- Smoked salmon (2 oz. thinly sliced)

What to Do
- Put all ingredients in a small bowl and combine. Add egg, water, and cream. Mix well with a fork.
- Add smoked salmon and combine well.
- Microwave on high 60 to 90 seconds. Once done, top with sour cream and enjoy.

Chive and Garlic Sunflower Seed Cheese

Makes enough for: 8
Time required for proper preparation: 5 minutes
Suggested cooking time: 0 minutes
Total required: 5 minutes

What to Use
- Chives (.5 c rough chopped)
- Lemon juice (.5 c)
- Salt (2 tsp.)
- Garlic (2 cloves)
- Extra virgin coconut oil (6 T)
- Sunflower seeds (2 c raw)

What to Do
- Soak sunflower seeds overnight in enough water so that they are covers with a tsp. of salt. Drain and rinse.
- Using a food processor, blend them up until smooth. Mix in the remaining ingredients and continue to blend until combined and smooth.
- Enjoy!

**This can be baked as well. Heat oven to 200F. Spread onto a lined baking sheet, or shape into a circle about .75-inch thick. Bake for about 45 minutes. The sides and top will be a bit firm, but it will still be very spreadable.

Avocado Hummus

Makes enough for: 4
Time required for proper preparation: 15 minutes
Suggested cooking time: 0 minutes
Total required: 15 minutes

What to Use
- Pepper (.25 tsp.)
- Salt (.5 tsp.)
- Cumin (5 tsp.)
- Pressed garlic (1 clove)
- Lemon juice (.5)
- Tahini (.25 c)
- Sunflower seeds (.25 c)
- Coconut oil (.5 c)
- Cilantro (.5 c)
- Avocados (3)

What to Do
- Halve the avocados, take out the pits, and spoon out the flesh.
- Place everything in a blender and mix until completely smooth.
- Add water, lemon juice, or oil if you need to loosen the mixture bit.

Zucchini Chips

Makes enough for: 4
Time required for proper preparation: 10 minutes
Suggested cooking time: 10 minutes
Total required: 20 minutes

What to Use
- Taco seasoning (1 T)
- Coconut oil (1.5 c)
- Salt (as desired)
- Large zucchini (1)

What to Do
- Use a mandolin to slice the zucchini into chip rounds. Place them in a colander in your sink and add a lot of salt. Allow this to sit for five minutes and then press the water out.
- Heat the oil to 350F. Working in batches, drop the zucchini chips in a fryer until golden brown. Set out on a paper towel and sprinkle with taco seasoning.

Stir Fried Baby Bok Choy

Makes enough for: 4
Time required for proper preparation: 5 minutes
Suggested cooking time: 5 minutes
Total required: 10 minutes

What to Use
- Bok choy (12)
- Sesame oil (1 T)
- Garlic powder (1 t)
- Coconut oil (1 T)

What to Do
- Wash and chop the bok choy into one half inch long pieces.
- Put the coconut oil in a frying pan or a skillet and melt it over high/medium heat.
- Once the coconut oil has melted, sauté the bok choy until it is tender and dark green. This will take approximately 3 to 5 minutes.
- Add the sesame oil and the garlic powder near the end of cooking.
- Remove the pan from the heat and serve the bok choy.

Spicy Riced Cauliflower

Makes enough for: 4
Time required for proper preparation: 5 minutes
Suggested cooking time: 5 minutes
Total required: 10 minutes

What to Use
- Salt (as desired)
- Chili powder (.25 t)
- Garlic powder (1 t)
- Bone broth (.25 c)
- Tomato sauce (.5 c)
- Coconut oil (1 T)
- Cauliflower rice (20 oz. freezer bag)

What to Do
- Heat the coconut oil in a frying pan over high heat.
- Add the cauliflower rice to the frying pan.
- In a bowl, combine the bone broth, the tomato sauce, the chili powder, and the garlic powder.
- Pour the mix into the frying pan with the cauliflower and mix it in well.
- Cook the combination for one minute longer, and then remove it from the heat source.
- Add salt as desired and serve.

Parmesan and Chive Mashed Cauliflower

Makes enough for: 4
Time required for proper preparation: 10 minutes
Suggested cooking time: 10 minutes
Total required: 20 minutes

What to Use
- Chives (.25 c)
- Parmesan cheese (.25 c grated)
- Chicken broth (2 c)
- Cauliflower (2 small heads, chopped)

What to Do
- Boil the cauliflower and the chicken broth for 10 minutes.
- Drain the cauliflower and blend it in a blender until it is smooth.
- Stir in the parmesan cheese and the chives. Add salt and Black pepper (as desired).
- The dish is ready to serve.

Cauliflower Fried Rice

Makes enough for: 6
Time required for proper preparation: 10 minutes
Suggested cooking time: 10 minutes
Total required: 20 minutes

What to Use
- Coconut aminos (5 T)
- Beaten egg (1)
- Onions (2 chopped)
- Sesame oil (2 T)
- Cauliflower (1 head halved)

What to Do
- Take out your Instant Pot and place a steam rack into the bottom of it. Add in a c of water as well.
- When that is ready, add in the cauliflower florets to your steam rack and place the lid tightly on top.
- Press your Steam button and adjust the time to go for seven minutes. When this time is up, do a quick release of the pressure.
- Take the cauliflower out and then clean up the Instant Pot to have it ready for later.
- Place your cauliflower into a food processor and pulse until it becomes grainy in texture.
- Turn the Instant Pot back on and heat up the oil. Stir in the onions until they are fragrant.
- Now add in the eggs, breaking them up into small pieces, along with the coconut aminos and the cauliflower rice.
- Adjust the seasonings as you would like them to be, and then serve this dish warm.

Chinese Eggplant

Makes enough for: 6
Time required for proper preparation: 15 minutes
Suggested cooking time: 5 hours
Total required: 5 hours and 15 minutes

What to Use
- Coconut oil (4 T)
- Garlic (3 cloves minced)
- Ginger (1 tsp. grated)
- Coconut aminos (.25 c.)
- Eggplant (2 sliced)

What to Do
- Take out the Instant Pot and get it all set up. Add in all the ingredients and season with some pepper and salt. You can add some more water if it's needed.
- After stirring a bit, close the lid and make sure it is on tight. Press your Slow Cook button.
- After 5 hours, the dish is done, and you can serve.

Gluten-Free Salmon Croquettes

Makes enough for: 6
Time required for proper preparation: 5 minutes
Suggested cooking time: 5 minutes
Total required: 10 minutes

What to Use
- Eggs (2 beaten, lightly)
- Large tin of red salmon (1 drained)
- Bread crumbs (1 c)
- Coconut oil (.3 c)
- Bunch of parsley (.5 roughly chopped)
- Black pepper (as desired)

What to Do
- Preheat air fryer to 200F. Mix together the salmon and mix with herbs, egg, and the seasoning.
- Mix together the bread crumbs and oil in another bowl until you get a loose mixture that can act as a glue for our croquettes. Shape the salmon mix into 16 small croquettes and coat them in the crumb mixture.
- In batches, put the croquettes in the basket and slide into the Air Fryer. Wait until golden brown.
- Serve.

Vegan Faux-Cheese and Macaroni

Makes enough for: 4
Time required for proper preparation: 20 minutes
Suggested cooking time: 60 minutes
Total required: 80 minutes

What's in it
- Onion powder (1 tsp.)
- Garlic powder (1 tsp.)
- Nutritional yeast (3 T)
- Red peppers (4 roasted, drained)
- Coconut oil (.3 c)
- Salt (as desired)
- Pepper (as desired)
- Lemon juice (.3 c)
- Cashews (1 c)
- Yellow onion (1 chopped)
- Coconut oil (1 T)
- Elbow macaroni (8 oz.)

What to Do
- Ensure your oven is preheated to 350F.
- Add a pinch of salt to a pot full of water before bringing the water to a boil. Mix in the macaroni and let it cook for 8 minutes until it reaches the desired toughness.
- Drain the macaroni and add it to a baking dish.
- Coat a pan in vegetable oil and place it on the stove above a burner that has been turned to medium heat. Add the onion and let it brown before adding it to the macaroni.
- Combine the salt, water, lemon juice, and cashews together in your food processor or blender and go nuts well. Mix in the onion powder, garlic powder, nutritional yeast, red pepper, and canola oil and process until extremely smooth.
- Mix everything together well in the baking dish before baking it in the oven for 45 minutes.
- Let cool for 15 minutes, serve and enjoy.

Chapter 9: Dessert Recipes

Berry Smoothie

Makes enough for: 1
Time required for proper preparation: 2 minutes
Suggested cooking time: 2 minutes
Total required: 4 minutes

What to Use
- Strawberries (.5 c)
- Raspberries (.5 c)
- Blackberries (.5 c)
- Ice (1 c)
- Apples (2 cored)

What to Do
- Mix everything together in a blender and puree until it has achieved the desired texture.

Apple–Rhubarb Popsicles

Makes enough for: 4
Time required for proper preparation: 25 minutes
Suggested cooking time: 0 minutes
Total required: 25 minutes

What to Use
- Rhubarb (2 c)
- Apples (2 cored)
- Ice (1 c)

What to Do
- Cut the rhubarb into pieces, the smaller the pieces, the smoother the results.
- Microwave the rhubarb until it becomes malleable.
- Blend everything until it becomes liquid.
- Pour the results into popsicle molds and let the results freeze
- Enjoy!

Baked Banana

Makes enough for: 1
Time required for proper preparation: 2 minutes
Suggested cooking time: 15 minutes
Total required: 17 minutes

What to Use
- Banana (1)
- Cinnamon (.5 tsp.)

What to Do
- Ensure your oven has been heated to 350F.
- Cut the banana in half lengthwise and then do so again before placing it on a baking sheet.
- Apply a light sprinkling of cinnamon.
- Let the banana bake for 15 minutes
- Enjoy!

Savory Nut Clusters

Makes enough for: 4
Time required for proper preparation: 10 minutes
Suggested cooking time: 10 minutes
Total required: 20 minutes

What to Use
- Salt (.5 tsp)
- Honey (2.5 T)
- Coconut oil (1 T)
- Raw almonds (2 c)
- Maple syrup (1 T)
- Cayenne pepper (.25 tsp)
- Red pepper flakes (1 tsp)

What to Do
- Prepare your oven by heating it to 350F.
- Using a mixing bowl, combine the honey, maple syrup, almonds, coconut oil, cayenne pepper, salt, and red pepper flakes and mix thoroughly to ensure the almonds are well coated.
- Add the almonds to a baking sheet that you have lined with parchment paper before placing the sheet into the oven for 10 minutes. Stir the almonds after 5 minutes to ensure they are well baked.
- Let the almonds cool for 20 minutes to give the glaze time to set prior to serving.

Vegan Cupcakes

Makes enough for: 12
Time required for proper preparation: 15 minutes
Suggested cooking time: 15 minutes
Total required: 30 minutes

What to Use

- Vanilla extract (1.25 tsp.)
- Coconut oil (.5 c)
- Salt (.5 tsp.)
- Baking soda (.5 tsp.)
- Baking powder (2 tsp.)
- Cane sugar (1 c)
- Flour (2 c)
- Almond milk (1.5 c)
- Apple cider vinegar (1 T)

What to Do

- Ensure your oven is heated to 350F.
- Grease enough muffin tins for 18 cakes.
- In a 2 c measuring c, add the apple cider and almond milk. Let it stand for approximately 5 minutes or until done, and the milk should have curdled.
- Combine the salt, baking soda, baking powder, sugar, and flour together in a large bowl.
- Separately, combine the vanilla, coconut oil and curdled almond milk in a small bowl.
- Add the two bowls together and stir well. Add the results to the muffin tins.
- Add the tins to the oven and let them bake for 15 minutes.
- Let the muffins cool before removing and serving.

Chocolate Peanut Fudge

Makes enough for: 12
Time required for proper preparation: 10 minutes
Suggested cooking time: 10 minutes
Total required: 20 minutes

What to Use
- Maple syrup (.75 c)
- Peanut Coconut oil (1 c)
- Chocolate chips (1 c Semi-sweet)

What to Do
- Add the peanut Coconut oil, maple syrup, and chocolate chips together in a double boiler turned to a mid-heat, stirring frequently.
- Add the results to a baking dish covered in parchment paper before placing the dish in the refrigerator and chilling overnight.
- Cut, serve and enjoy.

Chocolate Pudding Sans Dairy

Makes enough for: 4
Time required for proper preparation: 15 minutes
Suggested cooking time: 15 minutes
Total required: 30 minutes

What to Use
- Unsweetened cocoa powder (.25 c)
- Cane sugar (.25 c)
- Vanilla extract (.25 vanilla extract)
- Soy milk (1.5 c)
- Water (2 T)
- Cornstarch (3 T)

What to Do
- Mix the water and cornstarch together in a small bowl until it forms a paste.
- Add the cornstarch mixture, cocoa, sugar, vanilla, and soy milk together in a large saucepan.
- Add the saucepan to a burner turned to medium heat, frequently stirring to ensure it does not burn before it boils.
- Let the mixture thicken to a pudding consistency before removing the pan from the burner.
- Letting pudding cool for approximately 5 minutes or until done before refrigerating overnight to allow it to reach proper consistency.

Angel Food Cake Cookies

Makes enough for: 36
Time required for proper preparation: 10 minutes
Suggested cooking time: 10 minutes
Total required: 20 minutes

What to Use
- Coconut flakes (14 oz. sweetened, dried)
- Black cherry soda (.5 c diet)
- Vanilla extract (1 tsp.)
- Angel food cake mix (1 box)

What to Do
- Ensure your oven is heated to 350F.
- Cover a baking sheet with parchment paper.
- Combine the black cherry soda, vanilla, and cake mix together in a large bowl adding extra soda as needed to form a proper cake mixture. Once the right consistency has been achieved, mix in the coconut.
- Spoon the cookies onto the baking sheet so they are roughly 2 inches apart.
- Add the baking sheet to the oven and let the cookies bake for approximately 11 minutes.
- Add cookies to cooling rack prior to serving.

Orange and Anise Biscotti

Makes enough for: 36
Time required for proper preparation: 10 minutes
Suggested cooking time: 10 minutes
Total required: 20 minutes

What to Use
- Orange extract (1 tsp.)
- Coconut oil (2 T)
- Egg (1)
- Sugar (.5 c)
- Orange rind (1 tsp. grated)
- Anise seed (2 tsp.)
- Baking powder (2 tsp.)
- White flour (2.5 c)

What to Do
- Ensure your oven is heated to 350F.
- Cover a baking sheet with parchment paper.
- Combine the flour, baking powder, anise seed, and grated orange rind together in a large bowl and combine thoroughly.
- In a separate bowl, mix the oil and egg until the results froth.
- Combine the two bowls and mix well using a blender for 60 seconds.
- Roll the dough into a ball and cut the ball in half.
- Make each half into a long cylinder that is a foot long before flattening the top.
- Add the dough to the baking sheet and add the baking sheet to the oven before letting it bake for 15 minutes.
- Cut each cylinder into 18 equal pieces.
- Turn the cut portions of the dough so they are facing upward and bake for an additional 5 minutes. Bake the other side for approximately 5 minutes or until done and add the biscotti to a cooling rack prior to serving.

Sea Salt Almond Clusters

Makes enough for: 18
Time required for proper preparation: 20 minutes
Suggested cooking time: 10 minutes
Total required: 30 minutes

What to Use
- Sea salt (as desired)
- Almonds (2.5 c)
- semisweet vegan chocolate chips (12 oz.)
- Vanilla (1 tsp)

What to Do
- Place everything in your cooker and mix them together.
- Place on the lid and set to low for 30 minutes. Make sure you stir the mixture every 10 minutes. If you do not, the chocolate will burn and become stiff.
- Use an ice cream scoop and place dollops of the mixture on wax paper. Sprinkle the top with some sea salt. Place them in the fridge until firm. Enjoy

Berry-Choco-Cherry Snack Bars

Makes enough for: 12
Time required for proper preparation: 5 minutes
Suggested cooking time: 10 minutes
Total required: 15 minutes

What to Use
- Almonds (.5 c sliced)
- Chocolate protein powder (1 c)
- Pecan pieces (.5 c)
- Fresh cherries (.5 c pitted)
- Fresh blueberries (.25 c)
- Unsweetened coconut (.25 c shredded)
- Almond Coconut oil (.5 c)
- Coconut oil (.25 c)
- Almond meal (.25 c)
- Vanilla (1 tsp)
- Eggs (2 large)
- Salt (.5 tsp)
- Low-carb baking mix (.5 c)
- Splenda (2 packets)

What to Do
- Coconut oil a glass loaf pan.
- Set the oven to 325F.
- Mix everything except the fruit.
- Carefully fold the berries and cherries into the batter.
- Pour into the prepared pan.
- Bake approximately 11 minutes.
- Let cool for 10 minutes.
- Cut into 12 bars.
- Place into individual servings in snack-sized zip-lock bags.

Peanut Butter Bars

Makes enough for: 6
Time required for proper preparation: 30 minutes
Suggested cooking time: 5 minutes
Total required: 35 minutes

What to Use
- Cooked rice (1 c)
- Peanut Coconut oil (.25 c)
- Maple syrup (2 T)

What to Do
- Add the peanut Coconut oil to a bowl that can be microwaved before microwaving it for 45 seconds.
- Combine the maple syrup, rice and peanut Coconut oil in a small mixing bowl and mix well.
- Place the peanut Coconut oil mixture into an 8x8 glass container and then place the container in the refrigerator to harden for 30 minutes.
- Cut the bars and consume quickly when removed from the refrigerator to prevent the bars from melting.

Instant Pot Applesauce

Makes enough for: 4
Time required for proper preparation: 20 minutes
Suggested cooking time: 10 minutes
Total required: 30 minutes

What to Use
- Apples (12 cored, diced)
- Apple cider (.5 c)

What to Do
- Place the apples in the Instant Pot before adding in the apple cider, which will prevent the apples from getting too dry in the pot, which will ultimately make it easier to make them into a sauce.
- Cut holes out of a large piece of parchment paper such that it will fit over the inner rim of the Instant Pot and place it on top of the apples to ensure they retain as much heat as possible.
- Seal the lid on the Instant Pot, set it to manual and set the time to 10 minutes. Allow the pressure to release naturally when the time is up.
- Using an immersion blender, blend the apples until they reach your desired consistency.
- Pour the apple sauce into mason jars and cool prior to serving.

Peach Cobbler

Makes enough for: 4
Time required for proper preparation: 10 minutes
Suggested cooking time: 30 minutes
Total required: 40 minutes

What to Use
- Peaches (2 sliced thin)
- Baking soda (.25 tsp.)
- Baking powder (.25 tsp.)
- Fine sea salt (.25 tsp.)
- Cassava flour (.25 c)
- Goat's milk kefir (5 oz.)
- Liquid stevia (5 drops)
- Coconut flour (.25 c)
- Coconut oil (1 T)
- Vanilla extract (1 tsp.)
- Tapioca flour (.25 c)
- Egg (2)

What to Do
- Ensure your oven is heated to 350F.
- In a mixing bowl, beat the eggs, kefir, stevia, and vanilla together and mix well before adding in the coconut oil and whisking steadily to prevent it from solidifying.
- Mix in the baking soda, baking powder, sea salt, cassava flour, tapioca flour, and coconut flour and mix well. Whisk steadily until the batter is fully smooth.
- Add the results to a pie pan before placing half of the peaches into a single layer on top before seasoning with cinnamon.
- Place the pie tin in the oven for 30 minutes; you will know it is ready when you can stick a toothpick into the center of the pie and pull it out clean.
- Top with remaining peach slices prior to serving.

Vanilla Cakes

Makes enough for: 18
Time required for proper preparation: 10 minutes
Suggested cooking time: 15 minutes
Total required: 25 minutes

What to Use
- Vanilla extract (1.25 tsp)
- Coconut oil (.5 c warmed)
- Salt (.5 tsp)
- Baking soda (.5 tsp)
- Baking powder (2 tsp)
- Agave sweetener (1 c)
- Whole wheat flour (2 c)
- Almond milk (1.5 c)
- Apple cider vinegar (1 T)

What to Do
- Ensure your oven is set to 350F.
- Prepare two muffin pans (12 c) for use by greasing them.
- Add the apple cider vinegar into a measuring c that is large enough to hold at least 2 c. Add in the almond milk for a total of 1.5 c. Allow the results to curdle for approximately 5 minutes or until done.
- Combine the salt, baking soda, baking powder, sugar, and flour together in a large bowl and whisk well.
- Separately, combine the vanilla, coconut oil and curdled almond in its own bowl before combining the two bowls and blending well. Add the results to the muffin pans, dividing evenly.
- Place the muffin pans in the oven and let them cook for about 15 minutes. You will know they are ready when you can press down on the tops and have them spring back when pressed lightly.
- All the cake pans to cool on a wire rack before removing the cakes for the best results.

Vanilla Pound Cake

Makes enough for: 12
Time required for proper preparation: 15 minutes
Suggested cooking time: 60 minutes
Total required: 75 minutes

What to Use
- Whole wheat flour (1.75 c)
- Table salt (.25 tsp.)
- Baking powder (.75 tsp.)
- Sugar (1.3 c)
- Unsalted Coconut oil (3.5 T)
- Light cream cheese (8 oz.)
- Almond extract (1 tsp.)
- Vanilla extract (2.5 tsp.)
- Egg whites (3)
- Eggs (2)

What to Do
- Start by making sure your oven is heated to 350F.
- Prepare a loaf pan (9-inch) by spraying it with cooking spray.
- Whisk together the almond extract, vanilla extract, egg whites, and eggs in a small mixing bowl and set to one side.
- In a larger mixing bowl, beat together the coconut oil and cream cheese with the help of an electric mixer. Beat in the salt, baking powder and sugar until blended as well.
- Add in the egg mixture and flour slowly, starting and finishing with the flour and beat well.
- Add the batter to the loaf pan and bake for 60 minutes. You will know it is finished when you can stick a toothpick into the center and have it come out clean.
- Allow the cake to cool on a wire rack prior to serving.

Strawberry Shortcake

Makes enough for: 4
Time required for proper preparation: 15 minutes
Suggested cooking time: 0 minutes
Total required: 15 minutes

What to Use
- Low-calorie margarine (1 T)
- Semi-sweet chocolate chips (.25 c)
- Shortcake (2, 3-inch shortcakes quartered)
- Strawberries (12 hulled)

What to Do
- Using waxed paper, line a cookie sheet.
- Thread 2 shortcake pieces and 3 strawberries on 4 skewers.
- In a small saucepan, mix together the margarine and chocolate chips before placing the saucepan on the stove over a burner turned to low heat. Stir until the ingredients are well blended.
- Drizzle the chocolate onto the kabobs and then place them in the refrigerator for 4 minutes to cool.

Blueberry Snacks

Makes enough for: 16
Time required for proper preparation: 50 minutes
Suggested cooking time: 0 minutes
Total required: 50 minutes

What to Use
- Stevia (as desired)
- Coconut cream (.25 c)
- Cream cheese (4 oz. softened)
- Coconut oil (.75 c)
- Coconut oil (4 oz.)
- Blueberries (1 c)

What to Do
- Add the cream cheese, coconut cream, and berries into your food processor or blender and go nuts well.
- Add the coconut oil and the coconut oil to a saucepan before placing the pan on a burner turned to low heat and mix well as the coconut oil melts. Let cool 5 minutes prior to adding to the food processor.
- Process well before adding in the stevia and process again.
- Add the result to a pair of ice cube trays in 1 T serving sizes. Freeze 40 minutes prior to serving.

Strawberry Snacks

Makes enough for: 12
Time required for proper preparation: 10 minutes
Suggested cooking time: 40 minutes
Total required: 50 minutes

What to Use
- Stevia (as desired)
- Strawberries (3 diced)
- heavy cream (2 oz.)
- coconut oil (4 T)
- Coconut oil (4 T)

What to Do
- In an emersion blender, combine the heavy cream and the strawberries and blend well.
- Add the coconut oil to a microwave safe container and microwave it for 30 seconds before mixing in the stevia.
- Add all of the remaining ingredients to the blender and blend well.
- Add the result to a pair of ice cube trays in 1 T serving sizes. Freeze 40 minutes prior to serving.

Blackberry Cheesecake Smoothie

Makes enough for: 1
Time required for proper preparation: 5 minutes
Suggested cooking time: 0 minutes
Total required: 5 minutes

What to Use
- Ice cubes (6)
- Your choice of sweetener (as desired)
- Coconut milk (.75 c)
- Vanilla extract (.5 t)
- Coconut oil (1 T)
- Blackberries (.5 c frozen)
- Water (.5 c)
- Vanilla extract (.5 t)

What to Do
- Cream the coconut milk: This is a simple process. All you need to do is place the can of chill the coconut milk. The next morning, open the can and spoon out the coconut milk that has solidified. Don't shake the can before opening. Discard the liquids.
- Add everything, save the ice cubes, to the blender and blend on low speed until pureed. Thin with water as needed.
- Add in the ice cubes and blend until the smoothie reaches your desired consistency.

Orangesicle Smoothie

Makes enough for: 1
Time required for proper preparation: 5 minutes
Suggested cooking time: 0 minutes
Total required: 5 minutes

What to Use
- Ice cubes (6)
- Your choice of sweetener (as desired)
- Coconut milk (.75 c)
- Vanilla whey protein (1 scoop)
- Coconut oil (2 T)
- Plain skyr (2 oz.)
- Fresh orange juice (8 oz.)
- Carrot (2 oz. shredded)
- Mango (1 ripe)

What to Do
- Cream the coconut milk: This is a simple process. All you need to do is place the can of chill the coconut milk. The next morning, open the can and spoon out the coconut milk that has solidified. Don't shake the can before opening. Discard the liquids.
- Add everything, save the ice cubes, to the blender and blend on low speed until pureed. Thin with water as needed.

Vanilla Ice Cream Smoothie

Makes enough for 1
Time required for proper preparation: 5 minutes
Suggested cooking time: 0 minutes
Total required: 5 minutes

What to Use
- Ice cubes (6)
- Your choice of sweetener (as desired)
- Mascarpone (.5 c)
- Egg yolk (2)
- Coconut oil (1 T)
- Vanilla extract (.5 t)
- Whipped topping (1 oz.)

What to Do
- Add everything, save the ice cubes, to the blender and blend on low speed until pureed. Thin with water as needed.
- Add in the ice cubes and blend until the smoothie reaches your desired consistency.
- Top with whipped topping prior to serving.

Conclusion

Thanks for making it through to the end of the *Anti-inflammatory Cookbook 2021: Over 100 Delicious Recipes to Reduce Inflammation, Be Healthy and Feel Amazing*, let's hope it was informative and able to provide you with all of the tools you need to achieve your goals, whatever it is that they may be. Just because you've finished this book doesn't mean there is nothing left to learn on the topic, and expanding your horizons is the only way to find the mastery you seek.

Now that you have made it to the end of this book, you hopefully have an understanding of how to get started with the anti-inflammatory diet, as well as a recipe or two, or three, that you are anxious to try for the first time. Before you go ahead and start giving it your all, however, it is important that you have realistic expectations as to the level of success you should expect in the near future.

While it is perfectly true that some people experience serious success right out of the gate, it is an unfortunate fact of life that they are the exception rather than the rule. What this means is that you should expect to experience something of a learning curve, especially when you are first figuring out what works for you. This is perfectly normal, however, and if you persevere, you will come out the other side better because of it. Instead of getting your hopes up to an unrealistic degree, you should think of your time spent with the diet as a marathon rather than a sprint which means that slow and steady will win the race every single time.

Finally, if you found this book useful in any way, a review is always appreciated!

www.ingramcontent.com/pod-product-compliance
Lightning Source LLC
Chambersburg PA
CBHW080419030426
42335CB00020B/2506